SECRETS TO

EXPLORING FASTING AND A RAW PLANT-BASED
DIET, FOR HEALTH AND WEIGHT LOSS AS
INSPIRED BY THE ESSENES.

Florence W. Mabwa

First Published in Great Britain in 2018. Second edition 2019.

A catalog record for this book is available from the British Library.

ISBN: 978-1-68454-245-1

Cover Design by Faithbuilders | Cover Image © Ivdesign87 | Dreamstime.com

Contents

Acknowledgments

I want to express my appreciation to several people who informed me in one way or another in my journey of writing this book. Doctors and authors such as Prof A. Ehret, Dr. F. Bisci, Dr. L. Day, Dr. J. MacDougal, Dr. T. C. Campbel and Dr. C. Esselstyn, Dr. J. L. Ignaro, Dr. P. J. Adam, Annette Larkins, and Ernestine Shepherd. Although I never met them in person, they helped me define my thoughts through their great works and lives. Thanks to E. D. Szekely for writing such incredible books that have also greatly informed my path.

I also wish to acknowledge the painstaking editorial work of Laura Maisey, Mathew Bartlett and Jo Stockdale at Apostolos Publishing for their insightfulness, professional, and skillful work.

I want to thank my friends and associates who were a source of encouragement during the time of writing this book.

Finally, and not the least, I offer my profound expression of gratitude to my husband and children whose encouragement and patience have been indispensable for the completion of this book.

DISCLAIMER

The information in this book is for information only and is not intended to be used as a treatment for any illness, but to enhance your knowledge on how to better take care of your health. For all your medical needs, please consult your doctor or health adviser.

"If any man can convince me and bring home to me that I do not think, or act aright, gladly will I change; for I search after truth, by which man never yet was harmed. But he is harmed who abideth on, still in his deception and ignorance." Marcus Aurelius Antoninus, *The Art of Living Long*

"A man cannot have a better guide than himself, nor any physic (medicine) better than a regular life." Luigi Cornaro

Introduction: Why Should You Read This Book?

As a reader myself, I have read some great material on diet and health by several authors who have helped me on my journey to wellness. Books seem to be eternal in the sense that they speak even when the authors are gone. Some of the information that has helped me in my life was written over 2000 years ago, and it is still relevant today. So, having been supported so much by these books, I thought it worthwhile to write my work down for somebody else.

As one generation comes and goes, suffering the same fate of disease and illness, we feel moved with compassion. Is there a solution to human ills, a better way to live? Were we meant to be born, work hard like our parents, then die without notice from one disease or another? Our children take over from us, do the same things and eventually all suffer the same fate. I felt compelled to ask myself serious questions about wellness, and as you read further in this book, I share my questions and the answers I have found.

Human beings seem trapped in a world that is full of danger, and especially when it comes to the issue of our health, no one seems to be in total control. Doctors can help to alleviate the pain and suffering, but they too suffer from the same diseases.

I have seen many people lose their lives, some suddenly and others after much suffering. Losing people suddenly, without warning, from disease, not accident, left me wondering what life was all about. Why were we meant to suffer like this? Is there a way out?

As a Christian, I was even more concerned to know the answer. We all experience the same kind of physical suffering. I know that physical healing can take place through prayer, and I'm not discounting the life journey where faith is critical, BUT in this book, I ask the question: why are we experiencing so much sickness in the first place? I know our bodies are not eternal, and eventually, we must vacate them and allow them to go back to the earth, but I thought this should be at a ripe old age and with no sickness or pain. It should be a form of departure, a translation, like changing trains or a flight after happily finishing your work on Earth. Did our maker predestine this painful path for humanity?

It is true, and cannot be denied, that man must at last die, however careful with himself he may have been; but yet, I maintain, without sickness and great pain. (*Luigi Cornaro*)

When I began to struggle with these questions, I didn't know much about the effect of food and nutrition on our wellness. I had my own health issues (which I detail later), but I still could not find an answer. I asked myself why. Prayers didn't seem to relieve all the suffering either. However, I kept on searching for the correct medication and tried many options. Instead of my situation becoming better, it got worse! My body was becoming more of a problem for me as the years went by. And the apparent excuse we give ourselves is, one is getting older. People dread old age because of the many diseases and disabilities that are associated with that phase of life.

But in this book, I will explain how through my intense desire to know the truth I discovered some forgotten truths which many today have overlooked. When I made this discovery, I cried and wondered why somebody didn't pass this information to me earlier. I would have improved my health and probably never suffered any health issue.

When this truth was revealed to me, I wholly embraced it, and started a new journey. This truth became a guide for me, and since I'm still learning, I will continue to make it the basis of my new life. The transformation has not been easy. I'm still perfecting that which I've learned. Change is not easy. It takes time; but once you have the inner conviction, you will work towards your desired goal. Transformation takes a while, but as long as you tell yourself you want to change, you will succeed!

Many people reading this book are probably struggling like I was and would like some help. That's why I felt an urgent call within me to share my journey with you. I want to show you how to change your diet and lifestyle. I hope that somebody will be helped.

My desire is for people to be enlightened about the health choices they make. There is nothing new in this book but old truth being re-told again from my perspective.

If you are looking for ways to change your health, this book will help you discover the ancient natural ways to help heal and prevent diseases. It may be refreshing as well for those who are already knowledgeable and practicing some of the ideas mentioned in this book, to read about another person's experience of this method.

This book is a journey towards changing your **diet and lifestyle**. The optimum diet which we shall aim at is a raw **plant-based diet** that includes the option of raw, unpasteurized milk for those who want milk to contribute towards their healthy journey (even though according to many health gurus, dairy should be out of the equation).

My approach is informed mainly by the *Essene Gospel of Peace Book 1 with some parts of Book 4*, books which have been a fascinating read for me. This *Essene Gospel of Peace Book 1* has informed my healthy journey and continues to do so.

This book will discuss methods of fasting, which as we all know is a great way to restore us both spiritually and physically, and how this ancient procedure can help restore one's health. The enema is also an old method which some may not be familiar with since it is mainly used in hospitals.

I have discussed diseases such as cardiovascular diseases, thyroid problems, diabetes, cancer, acid reflux, Alopecia Universalis, and autoimmune diseases, etc., and the benefits for sufferers of adopting a healthy diet and lifestyle. Weight management is an area of interest for most of us, and I have discussed how one can lose and maintain a healthy weight. Finally, I have also included a summary of the Essenes diet.

I found the writings of Luigi Cornaro to be very interesting, and I have included some of his discourse in the book.

Writing this book has rekindled some of my childhood memories leading me to conclude with a beautiful poem to my mum who is no longer with us.

Chapter 1: Reasons for Change

"It is health that is real wealth and not pieces of gold and silver."

Mahatma Gandhi

I have always been fascinated with food and nutrition, but I had no idea of the "what's" and "how's." After graduating from high school, I joined a bank, eventually forming a career in financial services. Like most people in my generation the goal was to find a job and not necessarily in the area of your interest. As a youngster I dreamed of studying medicine and remained very interested in nutrition. In spite of the passing of time, my interest in health and nutrition remained strong, and it is this interest that has enabled me to write this book. I have been able to research and to read books and articles that would help me understand the relationship between the food we eat and our health. My search led me to many of the findings as we will see later in the book.

After losing some of my close siblings to heart-related diseases, many questions came to my mind. I was looking for answers, but they were not evident to me. Also, I suffered from a condition known as Alopecia Universalis which left me devastated for a long time. Other diseases of concern that affected me or some of my relatives or close friends included eczema, weight issues, acid reflux/GERD, thyroid issues, diabetes, rheumatism, and arthritis. Some of my relatives and friends have also lost battles to cancer. I have seen other people suffer from illnesses such as dementia, MS, and arthritis to mention but a few.

Reasons for Change

Though our health is essential to our well-being, productivity, and ability to fight diseases, it doesn't take a lot of money or time to achieve higher levels of health. What it does require is the right knowledge and a whole lot of determination. Getting proper knowledge sometimes involves time and deep thinking. Focusing on the outside appearance can be deceptive, and hence we need to seek complete health and wellness. Nothing in the human body operates in isolation. The tissues of our body are all connected via blood and nerves, and one's mind controls almost everything. There needs to be an agreement between our internal organs and our brain, as well as our emotions if wellness is to be achieved. The body is a machine or a house that is being driven by unseen powers within us. It is the failure to understand this connection that leads to problems. On the other hand, a failure to keep our bodies in a fit and healthy condition will inhibit the smooth operation of our thoughts and emotions.

My health journey was one of searching, seeking, and trying. It was all trial and error, and it took me many years to discover the truth. However, even after encountering the truth I was not immediately able to make a breakthrough due to deep-rooted beliefs systems and conditions.

As stated above, I had experienced many conditions which I had fully accepted as part of me. I came to realize that faith without responsibility doesn't work, and even if one gets healed, if there are no permanent changes to lifestyle, the illness may eventually return. No wonder Jesus, whenever he healed the sick, told them to "sin no more" (John 5:14).

It can be very offensive if you tell somebody that they are sick because they have sinned. "What sin?" they would ask. The reason is that we never consider things done against our bodies to be a sin.

> Do you not know that you are the temple of God and that the Spirit of God dwells in you? If anyone defiles the temple of God, God will destroy him. For the temple of God is holy, which temple you are. (*1 Corinthians 3:16–17 NKJV*)

Our bodies are temples of the Holy Spirit, and therefore when we misuse our bodies, we are sinning against our bodies. I guess the following can safely be considered sins against our bodies: gluttony, giving the body nutrient devoid foods, or the wrong form of nutrition, overfeeding or underfeeding, overworking or underworking, sexual irresponsibility leading to disease, etc. The body is just a vehicle and will do whatever we ask it to do, but that doesn't mean whatever we do is right. Eventually, the wrongs manifest themselves as sickness.

Since my youth, I struggled to keep my weight down. I had very little understanding of food science, and I denied myself nutrients to lose weight. I know now that my diet was devoid of high-quality nutrients such as those found in fruit and vegetables. I'm amazed at how long this went on, my many years of ignorant living. I grew up in a warm country, and perhaps this helped make up for other deficiencies that I would have otherwise faced. I genuinely believe that *"Man shall not live on bread alone,"* and that it was God's power that sustained me.

The pain of losing close family members to illness was immense and left me worried, vulnerable, and scared, primarily since the victims were not known to be sick before. Their loss has been a constant in my life, and I wondered in my mind repeatedly whether their diets could be blamed. On the other hand, people who ate the same food are still alive and well, and hence one wonders whether it is food or genetics that is at stake? I asked myself that question many times, so really, I couldn't convince myself or anyone that diet was to blame.

I would listen to researchers who would contradict each other about the health benefits of various diets. I decided to find my truth. It was during one of my periods of research that I encountered some fascinating information. It was my eureka moment. The knowledge I was looking for lay buried in a small book known as the *Essene Gospel of Peace Book 1*. From the time I encountered this book my life was revolutionized. I was transformed as far as my diet was concerned. I was like somebody who had discovered a great treasure. Many people argue about the origin of this text, but I received and accepted the information simply, and saw its power to change me.

Whatever we hear today from doctors, nutritionists, and diet specialists is nothing new. It is confirmation of a wonderful truth that was revealed over 2000 years ago. Unfortunately, this truth remains unknown to many people, but the time has come for us to embrace the truth regarding our bodies if we are going to escape the malaise facing humanity today. It's encouraging to see doctors, especially the ones who specialize in alternative medicine, nutritionists, and individuals through their own experience, finally receiving a wake-up call to this truth.

The Son of Man (Jesus) gave health to the sick, wisdom to the ignorant, and many other things, but details of his teaching on health and nutrition remained unknown until the information written in the *Essene Gospel of Peace* was retrieved from the secret archives of the Vatican.

I believe God is merciful, and the same Spirit that spoke through Jesus is again speaking today to many people who want to help themselves live healthy lives through good nutrition. However, it requires effort, obedience, and a good deal of heart-searching to achieve the transition to healthy eating.

The scriptures say you shall know the truth and the truth will set you free. But the truth is not only about when we leave this Earth; it is about how we should live on this Earth as well. Knowing the truth includes understanding that our bodies as temples of God's Spirit, and what is required to keep these temples in perfect order for their survival on Earth.

When our body is sick or is not strong enough, then it is unable to sustain the life that is within us, and we succumb to death. Of course, no one has the answer of how to prevent death, but there are things we can do to keep the temple healthy, strong, and durable. Eventually, the body will give way, and the soul/spirit will depart but this ought to be a transition rather than death, without sickness and pain after a right old age. At least that is what I believe God intended before men and women decided to go their own way.

In addition to the food which gives our bodies nutrition through chemical processes, we also need spiritual nourishment for our souls through prayer and meditation. Jesus said, "man shall not live by bread alone but by everything that proceeds from the mouth of the Lord," and so we should not rely on diet alone to overcome all the ailments and troubles of our bodies. A combination of the correct food and spiritual discipline will give us great results, and I hope that we shall be able to excel in both areas.

I have noticed that even when we observe good eating habits but are carrying heavy emotional burdens, these produce a kind of negative vibration as our bodies find it harder to overcome illness. Emotional healing is just as important as physical healing. The truth is, our bodies do not belong to us but to God. The body is a gift, or a vehicle loaned to us while on Earth to enable us to manifest God's image, but how wrong we are to imagine we can do whatever we want with our bodies and get away with it.

> We are builders of tomorrow, and we need not pay a fortune teller, a doctor, a lawyer, a preacher to tell us what will happen tomorrow … the inevitable will come, and we shall inherit the fruits of today's sowing. (*Dr. E. Howell*) [1]

However, we have a loving Father, the Almighty God, who cares for us and is concerned about us while we are on this Earth. He understands our predicaments and has made ways for us to overcome our problems. We must change our perspective and start to see the Almighty God as our Father who wants everything good for us. He is not there to judge or condemn us but to help us. He has given us enough information through writings, doctors, scientists, and ordinary people to help us. We need to obey and ask for strength from Him to enable us to walk in newness of life. Writing this book has exposed me to a lot of information, and I find it hard to believe that so many people are living in the victory while others are still walking in ignorance and darkness.

There are some who get the information but have no desire or ability respond to new knowledge. We advise clients to take life insurance when they are fit and healthy since that is the time to get a good deal. We take out cover then when we don't feel the need because if we waited until we were ill, it might be too late, or at least the protection we need may prove very expensive or even be denied. If you are reading this book and are in perfect health, NOW this is the time to start changing—you have no idea what is happening on the inside of you. Our immune system is very resilient, it fights diseases and illnesses, and sometimes you may never know what it has saved you from, but a time will come when it will be overwhelmed by the many years of assault and no longer able to cope. We need to support the body when we are in good health so that it remains active and operative for a long time.

Modern ignorance regarding the most important thing in life, the health of the body, is immense. But when people are sick, they realize that they have no worries about anything apart from their health. The famous Steve Jobs is reputed to have said on his deathbed that all the money he had earned could not buy him health. Apart perhaps from your faith, everything else: your money, self-image, fame, beauty, possessions, and all achievements become meaningless as you lie on your sick bed. For this reason, we need to get our priorities right and divest ourselves of irrelevant things. Our spirituality is affected by the wellness of our bodies while success and all worldly achievements seem meaningless when we lose our health.

The Essenes & The Essene Gospel

When I was searching for answers regarding my diet, I turned first to my Bible. I considered the Bible to be a spiritual book, but I was surprised to find some fascinating information regarding diet in Genesis 1:29 and Genesis 3:18b. Here, there is a clear guideline of what humanity's food is supposed to be. However, after the flood of Noah's time, there seems to have been a change in the original guidelines, and other foods were introduced. This left me asking, which was the best diet for me? The vegetarian-only menu of humanity before the flood, or the meat-eating which was permitted after it, as recorded in the book of Genesis, chapter 9.

To my great surprise, the answers I was looking for were written in the *Essene Gospel of Peace Book 1*. Some scholars refuse to accept the Essene Gospel to be true since they can't find its original manuscript and consider it the work of Edmond B. Szekely. If indeed it was, it was amazing how he came up with these details that have helped me and many others. He must have been a genius and really with such an illuminated mind. One only needs to read the reviews of many people to see how it has impacted their lives. For me, the information written in these books changed my way of eating, and it continues to do so. I had prayed for answers when I was at a crossroads. I was settled, and I have been since then, my spirit and soul echoed the sentiments of the blind man when Jesus healed him.

> So, they again called the man who was blind, and said to him, "Give God the glory! We know that this Man is a sinner." He answered and said, "Whether He is a sinner *or not* I do not know. One thing I know: that though I was blind, now I see. (*John 9:24–25 NKJV*)

So I don't know if the Essene Gospel is genuine—I only know it has produced genuine results in my life!

The Essenes

The origin of the Essene brotherhood is unknown. The Jewish historian Josephus records that the Essenes existed in large numbers, and thousands lived throughout Roman Judaea. They were fewer in number than the Pharisees and the Sadducees, the other two major sects in the time of Christ, but seem to have disappeared from history after the destruction of Jerusalem by the Romans in AD 70. Interest in the Essenes was renewed with the discovery of the Dead Sea Scrolls, which were likely documents recorded and stored by the Essenes.[2]

It is not so much that I have been fascinated by the Essenes as a group of people, though they were extraordinary and exciting in the way they lived. What interested me the most was the fact that they received some unique teachings from Jesus that I had not fully appreciated or understood before.

Some writers believe that Jesus may have known the Essenes, while others say he was one of them; for example:

> Yeshua grew up in the Essenes colony east of Mount Carmel where present-day Nazareth lies. Yeshua was the long-anticipated Messiah by the Essenes according to the order of Melchizedeki. He was called a Nazarene. (From the book *The Law of Light* by Lars Muhlmessiah)[3]

One can imagine that if Jesus grew up among the Essenes, then they may have had an opportunity to be taught by him on various aspects of healing, as he was one of their healers and a teacher of righteousness. The Essenes were a deeply spiritual group, perhaps because they received the teachings from Jesus. In other ways, they were not different from other Jews in believing the law of Moses and in God. The message you receive from these Gospels, especially Book 1 which is said to have come from Jesus, is spiritually profound, life-giving, fascinating, and liberating. It captures people's hearts. It gave me answers to some of the hidden questions that were in my mind. It was the vitality of these life-giving words that captured my imagination and set the path of change in my life.

Since this book is about a healthy lifestyle, I will major on the aspects of the Essene teaching.

The *Essene Gospel of Peace Book 1* is the most interesting and delightful little book. The author, Edmond B. Szekely, said he discovered original materials in the Vatican library of a manuscript written at the time of Christ or shortly after that. The book is about the healing miracles and general healing work of Jesus of Nazareth. Below is a brief extract:

> They sent out healers, and one of these was Jesus, the Essene. He walked among the sick and the troubled, and he brought them knowledge they needed to cure themselves. Some who followed Him wrote down what passed between Him and those who suffered and were heavy laden. The Elders of the brotherhood made poetry of the words and made unforgettable the story of the Healer of Men, the Good Shepherd, and when the time came at last for the Brothers to leave the desert and go to another place, the scrolls stayed as buried Sentinels, as forgotten guardians of eternal and living truth.[4]

Nevertheless, whenever I read his books especially Book 1 (he released the translation as a series of 4 books), I feel deep confirmation in my soul regarding the profound truths unveiled in them.

Until I read Szekely's books, I had wanted to change my diet but had not found convincing arguments to help me make my decision. But the *Essene Gospel of Peace Book 1* provides precisely the information I needed. It offers clear information on the advantages and disadvantages of specific diets and the consequences of the wrong choices.

The book resonated with me and I cried tears to know such truths had been hidden. My whole being received the information, and although I found it difficult to implement at first, with time I developed a gradual change. Regarding matters relating to health, I found the book very liberating. I was lost as far as my health was concerned; I had lost my hair, had weight problems, had arthritis problems, had lost siblings to heart-related diseases, and so many other health issues among friends and relatives. But the *Essene Gospel of Peace Book 1* has changed the way I do things. I later read the others books 2–4. I remember praying to God our Father in heaven, that if there was any information, some book out there that could help me in my journey, please would he bring it to my attention. I believe today that in answer to that prayer, so much has been revealed to me through the *Essene Gospel of Peace Book 1* and other writings that have been brought to my attention.

I find it incredible that this book—which may indeed have lain hidden in the secret archives of the Vatican for centuries—has given inspiration and has been a spiritual tool for over a million readers since Szekely first published it.

Chapter 2: The Hidden Cause of Diseases.

"Illnesses do not come upon us out of the blue. They are developed from small daily sins against nature. When enough sins have accumulated, illnesses will suddenly appear."

Hippocrates

We now know there are many diet and lifestyle-related diseases, such as heart disease, high blood pressure, type 2 diabetes, etc., which can be better controlled if one improves or changes their diet and lifestyle. However, we know some diseases are due to genetics and other factors, and hence it is true that not all conditions are affected by diet and lifestyle. Regardless of this fact, we have a responsibility to do what is in our power to do, to change those things that we can.

> If someone wishes for good health one must first ask oneself, if they are ready to do away with the reason for their illness, only then is it possible to help them. (*Hippocrates*)

Luigi Cornaro stated, "Illness does not happen without a cause, remove cause and illness disappears."[5]

I realize we are never willing, or sometimes we are unable, to do away with our adopted lifestyles even if we have a hunch that they could be causing us trouble. Sometimes due to lack of willpower or through ignorance, we refuse entirely to change until a severe illness sets in. It is never too easy to change one's lifestyle, but with determination one can make progress every day until the battle is won.

> It was never the intention nor in the plan of God to produce disease, but as logical consequence, through disobedience of the divine law of life, disease is produced. (*Professor Arnold Ehret*)[6]

> I cannot believe that God desires that man, his favorite creature should be in sickness, weakness, and sadness but rather that he should enjoy good health and be happy. Man, however, brings sickness and disease upon himself by reason, either of his ignorance or deliberate self-indulgence. (*Luigi Cornaro*)[7]

> The doctor of the future will give no medicine but will interest his patients in the care of the human frame, in diet and in the cause and prevention of disease. (*Thomas Edison*)

The following are some of the reasons why we might end up with deficiencies in our bodies:

- An inadequate diet that lacks essential nutrients. This occurs when we are not eating enough foods such as fruit and vegetables that are known to be loaded with many nutrients such as vitamins and minerals. However, the quality and freshness of these foods are crucial if they are to provide all that is required by our bodies. When we don't get enough sunshine, we run the risk of having shortages of vitamin D and all other benefits that we get from the sun. Cooking and cooking methods also reduce, alter or destroy the nutrients and denatures enzymes and protein. This may result in vitamin and/or mineral deficiency.
- Diseases and conditions such as Crohn's, celiac diseases and intestine permeability (leaky gut syndrome), may interfere with the body's ability to absorb all the nutrients it needs, and this may result in deficiencies even when someone is eating well.

In general terms, nutrition deficiency occurs when the body fails to get all the nutrients it requires to enable it to function well in all its areas of operation. Different vitamins and minerals are utilized to support different parts of the body. Most people try to overcome this kind of deficiency by adding supplements to their diets. Although this is helpful, getting nutrients from food is the best route, as explained later in this book.

How to Overcome Nutrition Deficiency

- Eating a balanced diet of fruits, vegetables, carbohydrates, proteins, and supply of good natural fats may support a healthy way of eating. When the majority of these foods are consumed in their raw form, the nutrients interact and become more beneficial to the body.
- Getting proper treatment for any known diseases such as Crohn's or celiac is very important to avoid long-term nutrient deficiency.

- With advice from your doctor, having supplements to help with any shortage in the body is sometimes helpful. For example, in some cold countries, many people are given vitamin D to offset the lack of exposure to the sun throughout the year. Vegetarians and vegans also are given vitamin B12, since this vitamin is mainly derived from animal products.

The following are some of the suggested symptoms of nutritional deficiencies: fatigue, weakness, hair loss, sleepiness, cravings, heart palpitations, poor concentration, etc. However, some deficiencies may manifest in different forms, and a diagnosis may be difficult.

Nutrition Overload

Arnold Ehret said, "Life is a tragedy of nutrition…. Man digs his grave with his knife and fork!"[8]

To survive on this Earth, we need to eat. Failure to feed our earthly bodies with food and liquids will cause them to emaciate and finally die. However, during our daily routine of feeding, we frequently put more into our body system than we require. When this happens, we end up with excess calories, and the body may store this extra energy as glycogen and triglycerides. If the body needs extra energy, it can obtain it from these stores. Carbohydrates are turned into glucose during digestion, and the increase in glucose in the blood leads to a release of insulin which in turn triggers the storage of glycogen in the muscle and liver cells. Glycogen gives the body an easily accessible source of energy for use in the brain, nervous system and muscles, especially during exercise. Carbohydrates are usually the best for increasing glycogen levels. If one continues to eat more and more without expending energy the body will convert the excess calories into triglycerides which are stored in fat cells. Most of the fats we eat become triglycerides. During exercise, if the body needs energy, it will get it from one of these three sources: glucose in the blood, glycogen in the muscles and liver, and triglycerides in the fat cells and in the form of free fatty acids. Blood sugar is the easiest way for the body to access energy, followed by glycogen. Fat takes longer to convert into the glucose that the body needs for energy.

According to the National Institute of Health, triglycerides are a potentially dangerous type of fat that is found in the blood. They are associated with various health conditions. If we continue to eat more calories than we need and still not utilize what is in storage, then the body will continue to look for room within the body to store fat. As a result, we continue to increase in weight.

Even though the food we take in may be "healthy," if it is continuously taken in excess then it will eventually cause trouble in our bodies. This scenario can only be rectified by taking drastic steps regarding our eating habits. One answer is to reduce the food portions we eat, to enable our bodies to start using up stored energy. This step can be combined with physical activity which utilizes the stored energy and eventually reduces fat stores. Fasting is also a great tool to help the body use the stored energy while it is rested from the inflow of food. Some people use the technique of intermittent fasting to curb weight gain by abstaining from food for several hours or days before eating. I think this is a beautiful method which enables the body to go back to its storage and make use of what is already there. But it must be approached with care to avoid creating health problems. People can lose weight on intermittent fasting, and more details on this type of fasting are given later in this book.

Toxins Accumulation

The term toxin was first used by organic chemist Ludwig Brieger (1849–1919). Toxins are waste products which can potentially harm body tissues. They can come either from within the body's cellular activities or from external sources including our food, drink, and the surrounding environment. Through normal body functions, less harmful substances are excreted from the body, but the body must work much harder to expel environmental toxins.

The primary sources of toxins are pesticides, antibiotics, and hormones. Others include packaging, house cleaners, detergents, food additives, pollution, heavy metals, etc.

If the body does not have enough essential nutrients, it will not be able to perform its normal function of expelling toxins, and the result will be an accumulation of them in the body. This accumulation, if not removed, may in time lead to illness, hormonal imbalance, impaired immune function, nutrition deficiency, skins problems, indigestion, fatigue, etc.[9]

Metabolic/Endogenous Toxins

These are toxins that are produced inside the body, some of which are waste products from normal metabolic activities. They are provided by the cells as they go about their normal metabolic operation. Microorganisms working on incompletely digested food in the digestive tract can also produce these toxins. Unless the body's health is severely compromised by illness or other conditions, then it is well equipped to eliminate these toxins from its organs. Most of the toxins that are stirred up from your cells are broken down in your liver and then removed from your body via your kidneys, colon, skin, lungs, and mucus linings in your nose and ears.

> Toxins become a challenge to our health when they accumulate to a point where they interfere with cellular function, a condition known as toxicosis.... While most chronic health challenges are caused by more than one factor, toxicosis can contribute to coronary artery disease, high blood pressure, type 2 diabetes mellitus, respiratory illness, kidney disease, liver dysfunction, autoimmune illness, hormonal imbalances, skin conditions, and most types of cancer. (*Dr. Ben Kim*)[10]

Environmental/ Exogenous Toxins

These include all the chemicals and pollutants that we get exposed to through food, water, and air. In general terms, an exogenous toxin is anything that damages the body and comes from food, the atmosphere, molds, heavy metals, pesticides, herbicides, prescription and over-the-counter medications, carbon monoxide, preservatives, food additives, pollutants, plastics, and other chemicals found in the environment. Toxins can be in the food we eat, the water we drink, the air we breathe and can be absorbed through our skin via everyday products such as moisturizers, soaps, and washing detergent.

In its daily purpose and functioning the body tries to preserve health, and when it's unable to remove all the toxins from the body, it may store the excess toxins in the fat tissues, then if the condition worsens it stores in other organs and tissues of the body.

If the body elimination mechanisms cannot keep up with the number of toxins that are coming in and being generated in your cells, then in an effort to preserve the body's health, the body will attempt to store some of the toxins in our fat tissues.

Our work is to support the body both by minimizing our exposure to environmental toxins and also by ensuring our nutrition and lifestyle remains healthy. If we do, the body will be able to clear out metabolic toxins and those that make their way into the system.

Some of the ways to naturally remove toxins from our body organs include:

- Drinking clean, pure water.
- Incorporating raw vegetable juice into your diet.
- A diet of fruit and vegetables.
- Exercising and stretching your body and deep breathing.
- Reducing stress and having enough rest to allow the body to detoxify itself.
- Losing fat through exercise.
- Fasting, as you will see later, is an excellent method to detoxify the body.
- Use of supplements such as chlorella, vitamin C, milk thistle, probiotics, etc.

Waste Accumulation

When the body is not able to eliminate the waste correctly from the system, whether due to constipation, lack of fiber, dehydration or other factors, toxins and unfriendly bacteria may build up in the body and if the condition persists, a disease may develop.

It is therefore crucial to ensure your body is properly eliminating waste products efficiently. The food one eats determines the effectiveness of this process. Whole fruits and vegetables in addition to other benefits they provide also provide digestive fiber which is crucial for proper elimination. In addition to fruit and vegetables, I found psyllium husk to be a beneficial addition to my diet and helps relieve constipation.

Acidosis

This condition, which occurs when your body fluids contain too much acid, can lead to many health issues if left unchecked. This condition occurs when the kidneys and lungs can't keep the body's pH in balance.

According to the American Association for Clinical Chemistry (AACC), acidosis is characterized by a pH of 7.35 or lower. Alkalosis is characterized by a pH level of 7.45 or higher.

There are two main types of acidosis. Namely respiratory and metabolic. Both can cause serious health issues. Respiratory acidosis, which starts in the lungs, occurs when there is too much carbon dioxide building up in the body due to conditions such as asthma and breathing difficulties, while metabolic acidosis occurs when the kidneys are unable to eliminate enough acids from the body. Types of metabolic acidosis include diabetic acidosis (due to lack of enough insulin in the blood) and hyperchloremic acidosis (can be caused by diarrhea or vomiting) and lactic acidosis. Lactic acidosis can be caused by various things such as prolonged exercise, prolonged lack of oxygen, cancer, seizures, heart failure, liver failure, and chronic alcohol use.[11]

Immune Deficiency

Immune deficiency is caused by the failure of the immune system to protect the body adequately from infection, due to the absence or insufficiency of some component process or substance. This disorder prevents your body from fighting infections and diseases and makes it easier for you to catch viruses and bacterial infection.

The immune system is comprised of the spleen, tonsils, lymph nodes, and bone marrow. Scientists say that these organs make and release lymphocytes. Lymphocytes are white blood cells classified as B-cells and T-cells. B- and T-cells fight invaders called antigens (bacteria, viruses, cancer cells, and parasites). B-cells release antibodies which are specific to the disease your body detects. T-cells destroy foreign or abnormal cells.

Inflammation Diseases and Lymphatic System Blockages

Inflammation is the body's natural response when it senses an internal problem, which may be real or false. It is one of the body's natural defenses against infections from bacteria, viruses, and other invaders. During inflammation, the body produces and sends white blood cells to remove and destroy any invaders in the bloodstream. Unfortunately, sometimes the body can trigger an inflammatory response without any real threat resulting in a condition known as an inflammatory disease. Inflammatory diseases will prompt the body to send an inflammatory response to an internal threat, even if no real risk exists. These white blood cells now have nowhere to go, and sometimes they can also act aggressively towards organs or other cells and tissue.

Symptoms of inflammatory disease include:

- Swelling of body parts, usually seen in the extremities, such as the legs, arms, feet, and hands. If they are not caused by external injuries, this can be due to inflammatory disease.
- Joint pain. Many types of joint pain are caused by inflammatory diseases, while different types of arthritis are thought to be due to inflammatory diseases, conditions such as rheumatoid arthritis, psoriatic arthritis, and gouty arthritis.[12]
- Stiffness and loss of function and movement in the affected area.
- Stomach and gastrointestinal issues. This can arise within the digestive system due to inflammation such as acid reflux, bloating, constipation and diarrhea. Type of diet and lifestyle can contribute to inflammation in the digestive system. A healthy weight together with an intake of fruits and vegetables, natural fats, seeds, starches, nuts, and proteins can contribute to overall health while it can help control inflammatory disease.
- Itchy skin. Skin inflammation may appear in forms such as rashes, skin itching, redness, and in chronic conditions such as eczema, dermatitis, rosacea, and psoriasis. It is therefore essential for somebody with these problems to be tested and treated for an inflammatory disease. Incorporating a healthy diet and a healthy lifestyle will help in the management of these conditions.

Treatment for an inflammatory disease can include:

- Medication.
- Rest.
- Exercise.

Lymphatic System Blockages

The lymphatic system is a system of thin tubes and lymph nodes that run throughout the body. It plays a role in:

- Fighting bacteria and other infections.
- Destroying old or abnormal cells, such as cancer cells.[13]

In other words, the lymphatic system is a network of tissues and organs that help rid the body of toxins, waste, and other unwanted materials. The primary function of the lymphatic system is to transport lymph, a fluid containing infection-fighting white blood cells, throughout the body.[14]

Organs involved in the lymphatic systems are lymph nodes, thymus, spleen, tonsils, and bone marrow.[15]

The most common diseases of the lymphatic system are enlargement of the lymph nodes (also known as lymphadenopathy), swelling due to lymph node blockage (also known as lymphedema) and cancers involving the lymphatic system, according to Dr. James Hamrick, chief of medical oncology and haematology at Kaiser Permanente in Atlanta.[16]

When bacteria are recognized in the lymph fluid, the lymph nodes make more infection-fighting white blood cells, which can cause swelling. The swollen nodes can sometimes be felt in the neck, underarms, and groin.[17]

In summary, the lymphatic system plays a significant role in ensuring the body is functioning correctly. It protects the body against outside threats, such as infections, bacteria, and cancer cells, while helping keep fluid levels in balance. One of the functions of this system is to drain excess fluid surrounding tissues and organs and return it to the blood. Returning lymph to the blood helps to maintain healthy blood volume and pressure. The body protects us from infection and illness by trapping microbes found in our tissues (mostly bacteria we pick up from the environment) and sending them to the lymph nodes, where they become "trapped." This keeps the bacteria from spreading and causing further problems like viruses. Once the bacteria are trapped, lymphocytes attack and kill the bacteria.

By adopting a healthy diet and lifestyle, we can help protect the complex series of crisscrossing lymphatic vessels. We also should seek medical intervention when necessary for correct diagnosis and advice.

Emotional Imbalance

Emotional imbalance mainly occurs when someone is not coping adequately with the things that are happening in their lives.

We all know that living a healthy lifestyle and having everything going our way doesn't stop us from becoming ill and dying of disease. They say money can't buy health, and we know this is true. Even access to the best diet and the best medical facilities cannot guarantee ultimate health for everyone.

Even so, the thoughts we entertain in our lives determine the course of our life-journey, hence the famous statement: *"As a man thinketh so is he."* In due time we must harvest the fruits of our thoughts and feelings, *the fruits of our free will.* Without knowing we allow thoughts and feelings of such things as fear, worry, rejection of self and others, unforgiveness, pride, hate, hurt, jealousy, judgment, criticism, dishonesty, immoral behaviors, inferiority and superiority complex to fill our minds. If you live and walk with these issues buried deep in your consciousness, they will influence who you are and what happens to you. But they were never meant to be part of you. Jesus said, *"Do to others what you would have them to do to you."* This truth works both ways, both positively and negatively. If you are giving out judgment, hatred, envy, etc., the same will be given back to you, and eventually, people can be overwhelmed by the harvest of their own planting.

In our journey we also experience trauma. We may suffer the loss of loved ones, illness or unemployment. We might separate from friends or face a divorce. Our children grow up differently from what we imagined and prayed that they would be; we may experience problems and not know what to do. Some people go into depression, and others contemplate suicide when they find their dreams are swept away. As age and disease catch up with us, we may start to wonder whether there is any hope. Most people have experienced one or more of these emotions because no one can escape the turmoil of life. However, a difference can be made by the way we learn to manage these emotions; how we offload them from our mind and heart.

Although on the outside you may look a healthy person you are sick on the inside, and no doctor can effectively help you. When you start to feel unwell the doctor will examine your physical body and probably ask you a few questions, but in most cases what they will treat are the symptoms, and the real cause of your trouble remains buried in your mind and heart. The body is merely manifesting the illness on the inside of you.

If you are seeking to achieve optimum health, I urge you to look for these hidden issues in your thoughts and feelings and try to deal with them even as you treat the physical body. It is vital that we balance our emotions for us to be in complete health. We sometimes give more attention to symptoms showing in our physical body when in reality the problem has its origin in our thoughts and our emotions.

> One who is injured ought not to return the injury, for on no account can it be right to do an injustice and it is not right to return an injury or to do evil to any man however much we have suffered from him. (*Socrates*)

Overcoming mental health challenges is not easy, and one needs to seek medical advice long before the situation becomes overwhelming. However, if one is able and willing, there are things you can do to help yourself. Feeding your body with nutrient-filled foods will help give you energy, and if this is followed up by exercise, this will enable your body to handle the situation better. If possible, identify your emotional pattern and be honest about your feelings—this is very important. Accepting the way you feel and look could be a step forward. There are many ways of supporting yourself during an emotional imbalance, but I acknowledge it is not easy. When I feel disconnected, I have found music very therapeutic together with prayer and meditation. If the situation doesn't improve then seek a health adviser or GP who may refer you to a counselor.

Stress

Stress is a way the body responds to any demand or experience, whether good or bad. When one feels stressed by something, the body reacts by releasing chemicals into the bloodstream which can give extra strength and energy. If there is physical danger, this would be a good thing, but if the response is due to an emotional disturbance, this can be a bad thing since there is no outlet for the extra strength and energy. If this is kept for too long, it will cause illness.

Chapter 3: How Fasting can Support Health Restoration

Why Restoration?

In the previous chapter, I discussed some of the root causes of disease, and in this chapter, I will address some of the ancient methods that have been used to help people get rid of toxins and accumulated waste while giving the body the support it needs to heal itself.

> Any man who is intelligent must, on considering that health is of the utmost value to human beings, have the personal understanding necessary to help himself in diseases, and be able to understand and to judge what physicians say and what they administer to his body, being versed in each of these matters to a degree reasonable for a layman possession. (*Hippocrates*)[18]

Going to see the doctor is critical, and we know they do an excellent service to humanity. However, it is essential for each person individually to try and support their bodies so that even the medication can work more effectively.

According to the *Essene Gospel of Peace Book 1*, some sick people asked Jesus, "If you know all things, tell us, why do we suffer from these grievous plagues? Why are we not whole like other men? Master heal us. We know that you have it in your power to heal all manner of disease."

Here I imagined a desperate group of very sick people, without hospitals and with very few doctors, and none of the medical science we have today. These people were impoverished. They wanted to be healed, and they were wondering, how did it become so bad for us, what did we do to deserve this? Can you help us, Jesus?

Regardless of medical advancement in today's world, people are still desperate, many with healing needs. When you visit Accident and Emergency departments, or hospital wards, you can't fail to hear the deep cries of the sick. These make me imagine the calls of the Essenes when they met Jesus. We all rush to A&E when something seems wrong with us, and we thank God for our doctors, nurses, and other health practitioners who help us in these difficult times. However, many questions remain which cannot always be answered. What is wrong with me? Why can't I be well like others? When we go to the hospital sometimes, we come home with some medication to help our conditions, and we are happy that at least something is being done about our situation.

When they saw Jesus, they wanted to be healed at once, for Him to touch them or say a word so that they would be cured. At least we know He did this on various occasions. Healing is what most of us want when we are sick. We go to the hospital to get the problem fixed, and we may also ask for prayer with an expectation that healing will come to us immediately, or at least soon. In the New Testament, we know that Jesus healed people instantly and they got well, but He also told them to "go and sin no more." The statement at least indicates that those who were healed needed to make some adjustments to keep their healing, even though it was not clear what kind of sin he was referring to.

In the *Essene Gospel of Peace Book 1*, Jesus gave those seeking healing more than they bargained for. What amazed me is that He didn't lay hands on them but instead taught and gave them a path to follow to attain good health. He wanted a permanent solution for them rather than a quick fix.

I have witnessed that most of the time the answers we seek do not come to us directly. If you ask God for financial provision, many times He will provide a way of you making money, a business opportunity or a job where you must do some work. I wondered why answers come this way. It seems that the Lord wants to provide permanent solutions instead of temporary ones. If God knows you will need finance, then instead of giving you £1000, he opens an opportunity for you to have a job, and a continuous supply of income. This can also be applied in our seeking for healing. It is good and necessary to find treatment from the doctors, and even ask for prayers when we are ill. However, if someone gets medication or is prayed for *but continues to do the same things that caused them to be sick in the first place*, their healing can only be temporary. Because of the love and care Jesus had for this group of people (and, I believe, for everyone today), He decided to help them using a route which was more difficult, but which nevertheless gave them a permanent solution. He also wanted to teach them a better way of living, but He had to demolish their wrong foundation and beliefs system first.

> Nor do they put new wine into old wineskins or else the wineskins break, the wine is spilled, and the wineskins are ruined. But they put new wine into new wineskins, and both are preserved. (Mathew 9:17)

And there is no doubt that if the one so advised were to act accordingly, he would avoid all sickness in the future because a well-regulated life removes the cause of diseases. (*Luigi Cornaro*)[19]

If someone wishes for good health one must first ask oneself, if they are ready to do away with the reason for their illness, only then is it possible to help them. (*Hippocrates*)[20]

In a nutshell, unless we understand what our bodies are and what they need to survive on Earth, our journey towards health may be a deluded one. We must understand the makeup of our bodies, and how to take care of them, just like we do for our cars.

The *Essene Gospel of Peace Book 1* says that Jesus taught the people about the laws of nature that need to be observed for the body to be in complete health. Imagine you are sick, and when you go to see the doctor, he first opens a book about human anatomy and starts to explain to you how those organs came about. Then he explains to you what happens when you put the food in your mouth and how finally the waste is expelled. Then he shows you how the blood flows through the arteries and veins and the type of food you need to keep yourself healthy and so on. Imagine doctors empowering their patients with such information when they are sick. I believe people would take their health far more seriously.

As mentioned in the *Essene Gospel of Peace Book 1*, Jesus wanted the people first to understand what they are made of and why it is important to treat their bodies differently. It was crucial for them to understand the Maker's prescription for their bodies, just like we read the manufacturer's notes when things go wrong with our machines. Without this knowledge, even today, we will continue to put the wrong fuel into our bodies. As we grow older, the effects of this wrong fuel start to show through all manner of problems and diseases. The Essenes were shocked to hear these teachings from Jesus, and I was equally shocked. I was shocked into action.

Fasting

The first recommendation Jesus gave to the Essene group was to fast or to renew themselves for 7 days before he could teach them how to take care of their bodies.

Renew yourselves and fast. For I tell you truly, that Satan and his plagues may only be cast out by fasting and by prayer…. For I tell you truly, except you fast, you shall never be freed from the power of Satan and from all diseases that come from Satan. Fast and pray fervently, seeking the power of the living God for your healing.[21]

From the above statement, we learn that fasting renews us. Fasting helps us get rid of the plagues or diseases that come from Satan.

It is not clear what method of fasting the Essenes used, or whether it included water, but many assume it was dry fasting. However, it is indeed beyond the scope of this book to recommend 7 days of dry fasting. Even 7-day water-only fasting is only safe if one consults their doctor to confirm their health status before they embark and if they listen to their bodies during the fasting.

Health is so necessary to all duties as well as to the pleasures of life that the crime of squandering it is greater than the folly. (*Luigi Cornaro*)[22]

Should a man when ill continue to eat the same amount as when in health he would surely die; while were he to eat more he would die all sooner for his natural powers already oppressed with sickness would thereby be burdened beyond endurance. (*Luigi Cornaro*)[23]

Why Fasting is Important

Spiritual Reasons

Fasting was a regular part of religious life in biblical days. Jesus fasted for 40 days before beginning his ministry. Moses and many of the prophets talked about fasting, and Jesus told his disciples and followers, "When you fast…." This reference shows that fasting was a standard way of life then.

If you will that the living God's word and his power may enter you, defile not your body and your spirit; for the body is the temple of the spirit, and the spirit is the temple of God. Purify, therefore, the temple, that the Lord of the temple may dwell therein and occupy a place that is worthy of him. (*Essene Gospel of Peace Book 1*)

Spiritually, fasting helps us to dislodge our attachment and love for food, and realize that we do not live by bread alone. When one keeps away from food for some time, the mind gets clearer, and one becomes more spiritually alert.

When we are freed from thinking about food and satisfying our hunger, we can turn our attention to feeding our mind and spirit. There are many spiritual blessings that we receive when we fast and pray. We are spiritually repositioned, and we can see things more clearly than before. Destinies can also be changed or shaped through prayer and fasting because our mind is calmed and able to direct requests to God and receive answers. Fasting gives us inner strength, and although our physical body may appear weary, the inner being is renewed. As we fast, pray and meditate our thoughts and feelings get freed from daily burdens. We fast to renew ourselves spiritually, to look through our lives and seek assistance from God to enable us to overcome the many issues we may be facing. Some of these issues are so deep-rooted that only the power of prayer and fasting can effectively dislodge them.

To be completely whole, our thoughts and feelings must be right as well as our bodies and fasting together with prayer and meditation helps us to achieve that. The mind, body, and spirit connection is the trifecta of health and to obtain real, vibrant health one must work on all three. Equally, the three parts of who we are must be aligned with the power of God. Our body is the temple of God's Spirit, and so needs to be kept pure. Fasting helps us purify the temple of the Spirit, so that the Lord of the temple may occupy a place that is worthy of Him. Spiritual fasting where prayers and meditation are carried out during this time helps us in this process of reclaiming the temple.

Many people fast for health or weight only, but they fail to understand that the body, soul, and spirit work together; they may partly achieve what they are seeking, but they miss out on the spiritual part which is crucial. Equally, others fast due to their spiritual needs but may fail to appreciate the health and physical benefits of fasting fully.

As you fast, ask God to set you free from the clutches of all that is affecting you, whether spiritual or physical. You may not be aware that you do some things because of an inside driving force, hidden evil powers which bring trouble to humans all the time.

There are hidden powers behind the many things we do that are not right and some that seem right but are only meant to chain us down. When you resist these powers through prayer, fasting, and meditation, you allow God's ability to help you get rid of them.

Health Reasons

> A healthy person has a has 1000 dreams, but when he has lost his health, he has but one.[24]

There are many people all over the world, religious or not, who have discovered the power of fasting as a benefit to their physical health. During a fast, the digestive system is rested, and instead of dealing with the inflow of current food, it starts to handle the work of repair, which it has probably kept pending for a long time. For energy, it will get a chance of using the stored glycogen and fat. This can only happen if you give it a chance through fasting. Any fasting will provide this benefit, although the speed at which this takes place depends on the kind of fasting, whether water, juice or liquid, partial or intermittent fasting.

> Instead of using medicine, rather, fast a day. (*Plutarch*)

> Fasting is the greatest remedy … the physician within. (*Philippus Paracelsus*)

Types of Fasting

Absolute or Dry Fasting

In this kind of fasting no food or water is taken for a set period of hours. Due to the many risks that this type of fasting would pose, I would not usually recommend it. However, dry fasting of 1–2 days with medical supervision may be tolerated by a few people. People who have managed to do so for short periods have reported amazing results.

Water Only Fasting

In this type of fasting only water is taken during the duration of the fasting. Since the bulk of the toxins in the body are stored in the fat reserves, the longer one fasts on water only, the more fat one will burn and the more toxins one will eliminate from their system.[25]

Liquid Fasting

This is a form of fasting whereby one takes liquids. The liquids may include, water, juices, teas, milk, etc. This is a very manageable form of fasting especially if one is still going to work or plans to have a long fast. The secret is to drink more water and have 1 or 2 cups of tea, herbal tea, 1 glass of fresh vegetable or fruit juice and more water.

Juice Fasting

This is a popular method of fasting usually taken to offer a medium of nutritional support in pure and natural form. If components of the juice are carefully selected, this type of fasting can give loads of benefits. However, it takes longer to get the same results you get from water-only fasting because the body will still have to deal with some form of metabolism at whatever level, which is not there in water-only fasting. They say this is the best, safest, and most effective method of fasting especially for those with health issues.

Although the old classic form of fasting was the pure water fast, most of the leading authorities on fasting today agree that juice fasting is far superior to the water fast. According to Dr. Rangar Berg (1873–1956), the world-famous authority on nutrition:

> During fasting, the body burns up and excretes huge amounts of *accumulated wastes*. It is suggested this cleansing process can be helped by drinking alkaline fresh juices from freshly made vegetables and fruit. Vitamins, minerals, enzymes, and trace elements in fresh raw vegetable and fruit juices are extremely beneficial in normalizing all the body processes during this time while supplying essential elements that may be useful for the body healing activity and cell regeneration. Though juice fasting is superior for healing and overall healing, it is said that water only fasting gives a faster form of healing.

Partial Fasting

This is a type of fasting where you significantly reduce food intake and only eat selectively for a set time. This works well for people on medication, those unable to get rest days, and maybe for people who want to fast for more days. A popular one of this type is Daniel's Fast (which is usually a 21-day fast with reduced and selected meal patterns).

Partial fasting is milder than absolute, water, liquid or juice fasting. It offers the same benefits of healing and cleansing of the body but the speed at which detox occurs, though more comfortable, is slower. It is a prevalent form of fasting especially for people who want to fast and still be actively engaged with their daily activities. I find partial fasting more difficult than water, juicing or liquid fasting. With water, juicing or liquid fasting, your mind doesn't think about food at all, especially after 3 days, and hence it is easier to manage in my opinion. It's easiest to break a fast with this kind of fasting because your mind is still thinking about food and checking on what to eat and what not to eat.

Intermittent Fasting

This type of fasting is currently very popular and is typically done purely for health and weight loss reasons though other benefits are also attributed to this type of fasting. This involves an individual staying without eating or eating very little for a number of hours (for example 16–24 hours). This can be done every other day or according to the plan until the desired results are achieved. The central idea behind the implementation of intermittent fasting is to reduce overall calorie consumption for weight loss by allowing the body to use the stored energy before receiving new food intake.

There is also the current popular intermittent fasting of 5:2 advocated by Dr. Michael Mosley.[26] In this type of fasting, one eats for five days, but for two days you take reduced calories (a quarter of the average daily calories). According to Dr. Mosley when one is going without food, the body takes the opportunity to get rid of old damaged cells and replace them with new ones, a form of cell autophagy.

Fasting Preparation

There are some methods of fasting which must be wholly condemned: irrational fasts, fasts without preparation, fasts of long duration without an experienced guide, and fasts which are only inspired by the wish to follow a system momentarily in vogue.[27]

Before a fast, it is essential to have a plan in place: decide what you are trying to achieve, both spiritually and physically. Reading the whole of this book before embarking on fasting will give you a deeper understanding of what needs to be done, especially in terms of diet before and after, including the onset of the healing crisis. Having a medical check-up that includes a full blood check, that includes essential mineral and vitamins being checked is very important. It is never advisable for pregnant mothers or children to fast.

Where one is experiencing nutrition deficiencies and still wants to fast, then vegetable and fruit juicing fasting, or partial fasting may be a better choice, but seek medical advice from a doctor before undertaking such fasting. Having a healthy diet that includes supplementation with important vitamins and minerals may be helpful before one starts a fast. Also limiting your food intake in the days before the fasting begins will prepare your body for fasting. Having a meal of fruit and vegetables for about 3 days before the fast is helpful to ensure things are moving in your digestive system and to avoid constipation.

It's very beneficial to do a fast during the warm season when you can go out in the sun and can have a walk outside for fresh air. This enhances the healing and elimination process as deep breathing is needed.

> When the organism fasts, it does not receive its customary source of energy from the body, so it is necessary to utilize other sources of energy; deep inhalations of sun irradiated air, which refreshes the nerves, pulmonary cells, and circulation of the blood. A large amount of oxygen introduced into the organism aids the oxidation of harmful waste products and increases the eliminative capacity of the lungs, thus preventing possible local accumulations of gas. (*Essene Science of Fasting*)[28]

It would be a good idea to plan to be off duty during the days you want to fast, for example, if you're going to take 7 days of water fasting as mentioned. The three days for preparation can be done while you are at work.

Though this is not possible for everyone, taking time off is beneficial because one can use that time to pray and meditate. For those with families, you still can create this time around your family if you prepare yourself well. Though fasting should be done secretly, letting some of the family members know that you won't be eating with them for some time would be helpful. They can also assist you in some of the tasks in case you are unable to do them.

Process

It's advisable to take laxatives such as herbal teas or enema when you begin fasting. This can be repeated when necessary. This will help in clearing your colon prior to a period of no food thus easing the fasting discomforts as waste is eliminated.

The first 3 days are the most difficult but from the 4th day the desire to eat may vanish, and this now gives one the best opportunity to pray, meditate, read, walk in the fresh air and out in the sun. We live in a busy world and having a quiet time where you seek God's presence, guidance, and peace is essential for our good health. When we spend time in prayer and meditation, we are trying to establish a connection with our real source of life, our Father in heaven, and when this happens, we receive peaceful and harmonious thoughts and feelings which can eventually be seen in our physical bodies. We may not be able to change our outside appearance, but we can influence our character and wellbeing with good thoughts, emotions, and actions. Prayer and meditation lead us to quietness and peace and give us the clarity and silence necessary for our welfare. In this secluded silent time, it is easier for one to hear or sense guidance in areas of your life. He will direct your path and will use various methods, it could be through the scriptures, through a song, a dream, a vision or an impression.

Perseverance and endurance will have to be your companions during these fasting days. When you focus on what you want to achieve other than the hunger, you will get the stamina to proceed.

> Many years have you yielded to the enticing of Satan…. And now you must repay them, and payment is difficult and hard. Be not, therefore, already impatient after the third day, like the prodigal son, but wait patiently for the seventh day which is sanctified by God, and then go with humble and obedient heart before the face of your Heavenly Father, that He may forgive you your sins and all your past debts. I tell you truly, your Heavenly Father loves you without end, for he also allows you to pay in seven days the debts of seven. *(Essene Gospel of Peace Book 1)*[29]

Depending on the condition of the body before fasting different people will experience different reactions. People may experience pain, coldness, hotness, and all manner of discomforts. Sometimes a lack of energy is also manifest. This is normal, but one just needs to be aware of it and adequately prepare to manage it. The first 3–4 days are the most difficult due to hunger, but after that, the hunger and desire for food may go. However, when the desire for food disappears the healing crises set in, in the form of pain and other discomforts. Accumulation of waste and toxins in the colon, stomach, and small intestine makes the first few days of fasting more taxing for the organism. You may experience headaches, heartburn, joint pains, and organ pains. Warm or cold baths may help relieve some of the conditions. Some days one feels great with a lot of energy, other times it's the opposite.

> You torment Satan with hunger, and so in his anger he torments you also. Fear not for I tell you Satan will be destroyed before your body is destroyed, for while you fast and pray the angels of God protect your body that Satan's power may not destroy you. And the anger of Satan is impotent against the angels of God. (*Essene Gospel of Peace Book 1*)[30]

How wonderful to know as you follow your fasting instructions correctly and though you may experience the healing crises, Satan's power over you is impotent against the angels of God.

When to Stop Fasting

> We must only fast up to the moment when the elimination of accumulated waste products and diseased cells is complete. We must always stop the fast at this point before the organism starts to exhaust its healthy cells and tissues, which are necessary for the vital functioning of the organism. (*Essene Science of Fasting*)[31]

Regardless of the set or aimed days of fasting, it's generally recommended that fasting should be stopped when true hunger returns (this can only be sensed if you are on water or juice fasting). True hunger is a sensation in the mouth and throat and not a gnawing pain in the stomach. This sensation comes typically after many days of experiencing no hunger. One suddenly has an intense desire for food. This may be a message that it is time to stop. However, a 7-day fast, especially if one is taking water, is a short fast and some people may not experience true hunger at this stage, depending on the condition of their bodies before the fasting.

This is a crucial stage to observe. There are several people who plan to fast for many days, but they stop before true hunger returns or when they experience other medical conditions. There are others who plan to fast for a few days but end up taking a longer fast because their bodies were able to carry on without a sense of real hunger. Being aware and watching for signs will be helpful and will ensure no accidents take place.

Finally, if nothing unusual happens during the time of your fasting then thank God and prepare to break your fasting on the 8th day.

Breaking the Fast

Just as I recommended 3 days preparation before the fast, so 3 days after the fast are also necessary to break the fast. On the first day after the fasting, one can start by taking soups, grape juice, or fruit juices and teas. The next 2 days should consist of fruits and raw vegetable juices, together with warms soups, etc. By the third day, your digestive system will be ready to receive some solids, but care is needed to avoid accidents.

Fasting Benefits

What happens during the fasting period is the most amazing thing and when you think of it, you get the strength to persevere. A lot of energy goes into the digestion process and so when we fast we lighten the burden of our weary and under-appreciated body. When we do not feed the organism, then those forces of the organism which are generally absorbed by the process of digestion are freed. Those parts of our organism which are usually paralyzed by the struggle against waste products introduced into the system and are customarily occupied with the elimination of excess and fermentations provoked by our irrational diet are freed from attending to the new foods for a while.

Whether fasting can help rid the body of waste build-up is a matter of controversy. However, fasting has been used for religious and spiritual purification for centuries.

Research tells us that even Hippocrates recommended fasting for his patients and used fasting as one of the methods of treating them.

Upton Sinclair (1878–1968) author of *The Fasting Cure* put it this way: "Those who have made a study of the fast explain its miracles in the following way: Superfluous nutriment is taken into the system and ferments, and the body is filled with a greater quantity of poisonous matter than the organs of elimination can handle. The result is the clogging of these organs and of the blood vessels." This, he says, is the cause of many ailments that the body experiences, so that, "The fast is to me the key to eternal youth, the secret of perfect and permanent health. I would not take anything in all the world for my knowledge of it. It is nature's safety-valve, automatic protection against disease ... it sets you a new standard of health."

Scientists say that when there is no incoming food, the organism begins to feed upon its own reserves and eliminate various old accumulations and deposits of waste products, which the body, while occupied with the daily influx of excess feeding, has no energy or time to do. This process is enabled during fasting. In view of all these useful physiological processes brought by a fast, fasting is considered an essential tool towards the healing of the physical and emotional body. Fasting kick-starts the body's own healing mechanism and enables the organism to heal from the inside out by helping burn the inferior cells and in building healthier cells and tissues.

> Fasting clears away the thousand little things which quickly accumulate and clutter the body, mind, and heart. It cuts through corrosion and renews our contract with God and Mother Earth. (Paul Bragg, *The Miracle of Fasting*)[32]

In short, some of the fasting results and benefits that have been mentioned in various pieces of research and which I have personally experienced include:

- Cleansing the body of metabolic waste and toxins.
- Stimulating new cell growth.
- Increasing mental awareness and energy.
- Resting the digestive system.
- Promoting inner stillness and meditation thereby enhancing the spiritual connection.
- Weight loss. This is one of the beautiful end products of fasting, whether one plans it or not. Depending on the diet one undertakes after fasting, the weight loss may be maintained, or it may all come back. One will gain some weight after fasting but not all if a changed diet is maintained.

Autophagy

This is the process by which cells degrade and recycle their components. Fasting helps by allowing this process to take place where cells can recycle themselves by dealing with the old and sick cells fast.

Dr. Otto Buchinger (1878–1966), the founder of the therapeutic fasting method, did not invent fasting but experienced it at a time when nothing else could help him. He described the entire process of fasting as burning rubbish, and he called it autolysis, refuse disposal.[33]

Autophagy is a natural regeneration process that occurs at a cellular level in the body, reducing the likelihood of contracting some diseases as well as prolonging lifespan. In 2016, Japanese scientist Yoshinori Ohsumi won the Nobel Prize for his discoveries into the mechanisms of autophagy.[34]

According to Dr. Eric Berg, autophagy is the process where the cells recycle damaged cell parts and get rid of pathogenic microbes, such as molds, fungi, bacteria, or viruses and everything else that is damaged and not working. During this process, they are sent to the liver for energy or get recycled as new tissues.[35]

Fasting has been used by many people and especially religious people for many years, but now the scientists are recommending it since they can understand its real benefits. I believe that fasting can encourage autophagy through a period of no food intake.

Though one may not fully understand the scientific explanation or benefits, we can experience the benefits fasting brings if we persevere and fast, not once, but regularly as Jesus said in Matthew 6:16–18:

> When you fast, do not look somber as the hypocrites do, for they disfigure their faces to show others they are fasting. Truly I tell you, they have received their reward in full. But when you fast, put oil on your head and wash your face, so that it will not be obvious to others that you are fasting, but only to your Father, who is unseen; and your Father, who sees what is done in secret, will reward you.

Fasting is, therefore, an ancient method of healing whose benefits have only been appreciated recently by scientists. Most fasters undertake to fast as a spiritual weapon and may not be conscious of the great miracle that is taking place inside the cells of their body.

Chapter 4: Enema

What is an Enema?

An enema is a fluid injected into the lower bowel by way of the rectum. The most frequent use of an enema is to relieve constipation or for bowel cleansing before a medical examination or procedure.

The purpose of the enema is to assist the lower colon in removing some of the old waste that has remained there for some time. Our colon retains so much waste even when there is a regular bowel movement. This situation can become worse during fasting because without enough food and fiber to increase the bulkiness; constipation may be the outcome. It is, therefore, crucial to have an enema before starting a fast and during the fasting period especially the first three days.

Colon

Our colon is the single most overlooked organ in our body. Even though Hippocrates said all diseases start at the gut, over 2000 years later, doctors, scientists, and researchers are just beginning to realize just how right he was.

Having a healthy colon is essential for digestive function, to be able to remove toxins and waste from the body so that they don't sit within the body and cause health issues. The colon along with the liver, kidneys and other eliminating organs—when healthy and in their best working condition—do a great job of removing toxins from the body. Bernado Lapallo who was a Brazilian-American centenarian noted for his diet/healthy lifestyle books, online seminars, etc., had a catchphrase "*Keep your liver and colon clean.*" He died of natural causes aged 114.

They say an average person has up to 20 pounds of undigested fecal matter (*poop!*) inside their gut, sitting there, just rotting and decaying. And if one has leaky gut syndrome, this toxic fecal matter leaks through the gut wall into the bloodstream contributing to many health issues.

> I tell you truly, the uncleanness within is greater by much than the uncleanness without. And he who cleanses himself without, but within remains unclean, is like tombs that outwards are painted fair, but are within full of all manner of horrible uncleanness and abominations. (*Essene Gospel of Peace Book 1*)[36]

When we are fasting a lot of harmful waste products, loaded with toxins, enter the intestines and stay there. It is best if these toxic materials can be eliminated as soon as possible to prevent fermentation that would cause more pressure on the colon and nervous system. When we eat food with the right amount of fiber, vegetables, and fruit, our colon can eliminate waste faster and more efficiently. However, during fasting where food is either reduced or stopped altogether the waste may be retained in the system for longer and that is why we have talked about the need to *prepare* before undertaking the fast.

An enema used during the first few days of fasting helps the colon to undertake this task with more comfort when there isn't much fiber to assist. For better success with colon cleaning it is good to extend this help also to the stomach and small intestine. This can be done by drinking plenty of water, fresh lemon juice with some honey, herbal teas, and psyllium husk may help move things before an enema is done. Diets with enough vegetables and fruit should be taken every day if one is not fasting to help the colon. When we don't combine an enema with fasting, all these toxic materials and waste are left in the colon, and the body must make some effort to get rid of them by the normal process of excretion. It is not common today for people to perform enemas. Neither did I until I read the *Essene Gospel of Peace*. It was through reading this that I learned how to use an enema as a supportive tool. In my research, I discovered that enemas were widely used as a health-supporting tool in the olden days and even Hippocrates used it to treat his patients. The primary goal of an enema is not to interfere with digestion but to help/support the colon in removing the accumulated waste.

Though ideally an enema should be performed by trained people, it can be self-administered. *It's important to seek medical advice from health professionals before you decide to do it.* An enema should not be done without proper research and training. This book is for information only and is not meant to be taken as medical advice. My aim is to raise awareness for those who may not be aware of this ancient method that is still widely used by people all over the world. I was ignorant of the kind of waste our colon/bowels are subjected to due to poor choices of food and lifestyle. Though the body can perform this process without interference, unfortunately, due to the kind of diet we eat (both the type and amount of food we choose) the colon continuously holds waste and sometimes for too long before it's properly eliminated out of the body.

The kind of enema that was recommended to the Essenes was with pure water with nothing added, and it was mainly administered to the sick to help them recover from illnesses. Other similar types of enemas include colonics and coffee or wheatgrass enemas etc. If one wants to learn more on this, there is a lot of information out there and in places such as Gerson Institute or Gerson Therapy.[37]

To ensure that an enema does not cause a gut-flora imbalance, severe dehydration, and electrolyte imbalance, it is advisable to use probiotics and to drink at least 6–8 glasses of water supplemented with essential electrolytes such as sodium, potassium, calcium, bicarbonate, magnesium, chloride and phosphate when necessary.

Disclaimer—Please seek medical professional advice and guidance if you want to perform an enema at home.

Chapter 5: How to Restore your Health with Changed Diet and Lifestyle

After a successful fasting period of 7 days, one will experience significant changes both physically and spiritually. The positive results may take some time to manifest. However, what we do and what we eat after fasting will determine our eventual success. For many years we have given our body the wrong kind of fuel, and now we have restarted the machine through prayer and fasting. Now at this stage, we want to go back to the manufacturer's manual and see what He intended us to fuel our bodies with.

Recovery is an individual task, and no doctor can really restore your health if you are not willing to bring about changes in your life. It is very easy to go back to your old way of living again, and that is why planning ahead is crucial.

> The doctor of the future will give no medicine but will interest his patients in the care of the human frame, in diet and in the cause and prevention of disease. (*Thomas Edison*)

> Whenever we follow the path of reason, everything will be satisfactory, but as soon as we deviate from the path of reason, everything in life goes wrong. (*Socrates*)

Going Back to Basics

> And God said, "See, I have given you every **herb *that* yields seed** which *is* on the face of all the Earth, and every **tree whose fruit yields seed**; to you it shall be for food. Also, to every beast of the Earth, to every bird of the air, and to everything that creeps on the Earth, in which *there is* life, *I have given* **every green herb for food**"; and it was so. (Genesis 1:29–30)

> Behold, I have given you every **herb bearing seed**, which is upon the face of all the Earth, and every tree, in which is **the fruit** of a tree yielding seed; to you it shall be for meat. And to every beast of the Earth, and to every fowl of the air, and to everything that creeps upon the Earth, wherein there is the breath of life, I give every green herb for meat. Also, **the milk of everything (beasts) that moves** and lives upon Earth shall be meat for you; even as the **green herbs** have, I

have given unto them, so I give **their milk** unto you. *(Essene Gospel of Peace Book 1)*[38]

So, eat always from the table of God, the fruits of the tree, the grains and grasses (this include all grass, all trees, and all plants in every part of the world) of the field, the milk of the beast and the honey of bees. *(Essene Gospel of Peace Book 1)*[39]

The original food groups of humanity from the beginning:

- Fruits—such as apples, mangoes, all berries, pineapples, pears, peaches, oranges, nectarines, grapes, etc.
- Grains—such as wheat, millet, oats, corn, rice, barley, quinoa, buckwheat, and amaranth, etc.
- Grasses of the field—herbs, vegetables, all plants good for food are in this group.
- Milk of the beast—such as goats, sheep and cows' milk. We shall, however, see how man himself has changed the milk and its production hence causing all the troubles associated with milk today.
- Honey of bees—raw organic honey.

Why Fruits of the Trees?

Everyone knows the benefit of fruits, as they are the best foods that need no cooking, are deliciously tasty, with many varieties to choose from in a range of attractive colors.

Fruit and vegetables are a good source of vitamins and minerals, including folate, vitamin C, and potassium. They're an excellent source of dietary fiber, which can help to maintain a healthy gut and prevent constipation and other digestion problems. A diet high in fiber can also reduce your risk of bowel cancer.

Why Grains?

Most known and used grains include wheat, millet, oats, corn, rice barley, quinoa, buckwheat, amaranth, etc. These grains eaten whole will provide energy and nutrients to our bodies. They form part of complex starches which are needed to help us eat a balanced diet. Grains have been used all over the world as a staple food and honestly grains consumed in the right portions and without adding oil do not add weight. They are an essential part of diet since they give energy that the body needs for its daily activity. In different parts of developing countries, the following are used on a regular basis as food: rice, corn (maize), millet, wheat, sorghum, etc. Most of the grains, especially the dry ones, are seeds in a dormant stage, and it is important to sprout (germinate) them to add nutritional value and reduce adverse effects.

Sprouting is essentially the practice of germinating seeds, whether grains, nuts, beans or other kinds of seed. Some of the benefits of sprouting according to Dr. Axe are:

- Sprouting increases the nutrient absorption of vitamins and minerals such as B12, iron, magnesium, and zinc.
- Sprouting makes food easier to digest because it helps to release enzymes that make it easier for the digestive system.
- It helps decrease some anti-nutrients and phytic acid.
- Increases proteins availability.
- Increases fiber content.
- Breaks down gluten for easier digestion.
- Helps reduce other allergens found in grains and legumes.
- May increase enzymes and antioxidants.[40]

Some Basic Truths about Food

The following shows the calories we get from each food group per gram as shown in various sources:

> Fat: 1 gram = 9 calories.
> Protein: 1 gram = 4 calories.
> Carbohydrates: 1 gram = 4 calories.
> Alcohol: 1 gram = 7 calories.[41]

The above information is crucial because most people omit carbohydrates from their meals in the belief that they contribute a high number of calories to their diet—which you can see from the above table is not the case. Carbohydrates usually add weight only because of added fat and sugar.

The primary nutrients found in food that provide energy are protein, fat, and carbohydrates and it is crucial to understand the sources of these and the way you should eat them to have a balanced diet.

Plants (Grasses) of the Field

This includes all vegetables and plants that are edible and can be used as food. The grasses include the greens (the leaves) but also root vegetables, grains, and seeds. The importance of eating green vegetables and particularly leafy green vegetables has been frequently highlighted, though sometimes we don't stop to think why this is so. What is so special about green vegetables? Aren't all the vegetables the same?

The reason why green, particularly green leafy vegetables are a superfood is because of their chlorophyll content, which is very important as part of the healing of the body.

> Fruit trees of all kinds will grow along both sides of the river. The leaves of these trees will never turn brown and fall, and there will always be fruit on their branches. There will be a new crop every month, for they are watered by the river flowing from the Temple. The fruit will be for food and the leaves for healing. (Ezekiel 47:12 NLT)

The Power of the Green in Plants

Dark green leafy vegetables are excellent sources of nutrition. Salad greens, kale, and spinach are rich in vitamins A, C, E and K, and broccoli, bok choy and mustard are also rich in many of the B-vitamins. These vegetables also contain an abundance of carotenoids-antioxidants that protect cells and play roles in blocking the early stages of cancer. They also provide high levels of fiber, iron, magnesium, potassium, and calcium. Furthermore, greens have minimal carbohydrates, sodium, and cholesterol. The dark greens supply a significant amount of folate, a B vitamin that promotes heart health.[42]

Because of their high content of antioxidants, green leafy vegetables may be one of the best health-supporting foods. Another benefit of eating dark green leafy vegetables is the fact that they are low in calories and hence are useful for maintaining healthy body weight.

Green vegetables contain large amounts of a green pigment called chlorophyll. Chlorophyll helps plants convert sunlight into energy in a process called photosynthesis. But chlorophyll isn't just good for plants; it's good for humans too.[43]

What is Chlorophyll?

Chlorophyll is the molecule in plants that absorbs sunlight and uses its energy to synthesize carbohydrates from CO_2 and water. This process is known as photosynthesis and is the basis for sustaining the life processes of all plants. Since animals and humans obtain their food supply by eating plants, photosynthesis can be said to be the source of our life also.[44]

The above scientific explanation of the chlorophyll (the green color) is fascinating. In the *Essene Gospel*, Jesus talks about the gift of life that is in the grass; the grass here represents all plants, as you have read. It's amazing how the color green comes about—the plant is able to "catch" the power of the sun in the light. Using wheatgrass as an example, Jesus *said: "in the tender grass lies the secrets of all angels, angels of the sun give green color to the grass."* That is, chlorophyll absorbs light from the sun to make energy in plants, and it's this that gives plants their green color.

> I tell you the truth all that is green and with life has the power of the angel of the sun within it…. For I tell you since no one can look upon the sun when it is shining in the heavens because of its radiant light. The angel of the sun, therefore, turns the grass green and all that she gives life, that man may look upon many and various shades of green and find strength and comfort therein…. Truly it is not only as bread that wheat may nourish us; we may also eat of the tender blades of grass (wheatgrass) that God's power may enter us. (*Essene Gospel of Peace, Book 4, 270–273*)

Nature has put itself the problem of how to catch light streaming to the Earth and to store the most elusive of all powers in rigid form. The plants take in one kind of energy, light; and produce another energy, chemical difference.[45]

The best sources of chlorophyll found on the planet are green vegetables and algae. One of the primary ways of including chlorophyll in the diet is by eating green vegetables. Top sources include leafy green vegetables such as kale, spinach, swiss chard, watercress, peas, artichoke, broccoli, bok choy, asparagus, etc., and algae such as chlorella and spirulina. Chlorophyll content is decreased when green vegetables are cooked, and hence most of these vegetables are best eaten raw. There are chlorophyll supplements in the market, some in liquid form, though the best source would be fresh raw green vegetables or a green vegetable juice. Green juice is currently widely used all over the world.

Raw Honey

Honey is one of the foods we were given in creation. I keep wondering, "why?" Most of us like honey though we are always conscious about its sugar content. Honey is used widely all over the world and as an ingredient in many products. However, just as in the case of milk (to be discussed later), most of the honey out there is not pure honey, it is pasteurized/heated to kill harmful bacteria and then processed, often with added sugar.

However, unlike raw milk, it's easy to get raw honey in many supermarkets and health stores. Raw honey is more expensive and has fewer suppliers. Raw honey, just like raw milk, needs to be sourced from reputable suppliers to ensure no contamination that would cause illness. All foods carry the risk of harmful bacteria, something that is true even when they are correctly and organically sourced. Milk can carry bacteria from the cow or goat. Vegetables can carry harmful bacteria from the soil or insects. Harmful bacteria can also find their way into food during transportation, distribution, and storage. The killing of harmful bacteria is one reason that makes pasteurization of milk and even honey attractive, but as you will read in the next chapter, this is not without cost.

Honey has many health benefits if used sparingly and in moderation. Honey is alkaline when eaten raw but *is about 55 percent fructose, a fruit sugar that's processed by the liver.*

Despite the chemical difference, our bodies still react to honey in much the same way as they respond to refined sugar, with a blood-sugar spike which encourages the pancreas to produce insulin and may lead the body to store fat with an eventual weight gain if taken in excess.

Raw honey is beneficial food and can be used instead of refined sugar. People use honey for mild medicinal solutions such as colds, coughs, indigestion, and constipation. However, due to the possibility of spores of Clostridium botulinum bacteria in some honey, it's not advisable to feed honey to infants.

Some of the stated benefits of honey are as follows:

- Reduces cough and throat irritation, powerful decongestant.
- Heals wounds and burns.

- Acts as anti-bacterial, anti-microbial and anti-fungal.
- Reduces ulcers and other gastrointestinal disorder.
- Honey is said to contain friendly bacteria.

Milk

Milk has been mentioned as one of the foods that were given to humans. However, the diverse opinions on the health pros and cons of milk are very confusing. In spite of the negative publicity, milk is still a very popular drink all over the world. Vegans don't take milk purely because it's an animal product while others are milk intolerant and this is understandable. However, currently, there is a big group of studies that indicate milk is bad for our health. How could a drink that is so popular be bad for our health? Some dairy products are also blamed as contributing factors in cardiovascular disease, because of the saturated fat in the milk that contributes to LDL (bad) cholesterol and clogging of the arteries.

Milk is a widely used product all over the world and is mentioned in the *Essene Gospel of Peace Book 1* as one of the foods that God gave to man.

> And in the month of Tevet (December) begin to eat also the milk of your beasts, because after this did the Lord give the herbs of the fields to all the beasts which render milk that they might with their milk feed man. (*Essene Gospel of Peace Book 1*)[46]

This is an amazing statement, clearly showing that God designed for animals to feed humans with their milk. Milk has been used all over the world to help young babies and children meet their nutrition balance (though currently there are a few people who do not advocate this). Whole communities take milk as a staple food. If you have any allergic reaction when you drink milk, try other types of milk such as goats' milk. There are many other milk substitutes, too, from vegetable sources, if you are unable to take animal milk.

What Happens to Milk?

Raw milk can harbor large amounts of pathogenic organisms such as Brucella, Campylobacter, Listeria, and other bacteria that can lead to sickness, sometimes severe illness, especially in the very young and the elderly.

Some of the contamination from milk comes from the environment in which animals are being milked, in the processing, storage, and delivery. If the animals are sick, for example, with diseases like tuberculosis, then contamination can (rarely) come from within the animal. Other sources of contamination can be the bacteria that live on the animal's skin or an infection of the udders (mastitis). Milk producers themselves can contribute to contamination if proper hygiene is not observed.

The kind of milk that God gave to humans is not the same kind of milk that most farmers produce today. Due to the high demand and the desire to profit man has gone to the pervasive measures to cause the "beasts" to over-produce the milk and to make it available all the time. A lot has happened to alter the original cow to the present one to increase milk production. When it comes to feeding the animals, humans also have interfered with this crucial stage; the animals were meant to eat the grasses and green herbs and all-natural fresh plants to produce nutritious milk. But in many areas, milk-producing animals are fed hormonal foods, so that milk production is consistent and plentiful, but not natural. Too little concern is placed on nutritional content and the long-term effects of these actions. We have mentioned before the benefits of the chlorophyll that comes from the green plants. When animals feed on grass and herbs that are full of these benefits, they eventually pass these benefits to humans through their milk.

Thankfully, many farmers today allow their animals to feed on grass and herbs and their milk is produced organically, and the animals move freely in the farm to graze on grass.

Once the milk has been produced by the animals, whether organic or not, it is passed through another stage before it becomes available at the stores. At this stage, the milk is heated to high temperatures, a process known as pasteurization. Pasteurization kills germs, bacteria, and pathogens in the milk, and lengthens the shelf-life of the milk.

Chapter 6: Pasteurization

What is Pasteurization?

Pasteurization is a process that kills harmful bacteria by heating milk to a specific temperature for a set period of time (72°c [161°f] for 15 seconds; UHT is heated at 140°c [284°f] for four seconds). First developed by Louis Pasteur in 1864, pasteurization kills harmful organisms responsible for such diseases as listeriosis, typhoid fever, tuberculosis, diphtheria, and brucellosis.[47]

Why Pasteurization?

The idea of having pasteurized milk was to increase safety and preservation. To protect people from diseases caused by milk contamination during production and distribution, most countries allow only pasteurized milk. In some states, raw milk is also available but not enough to meet the demands of the people.

Unfortunately, this process also ended up altering one of the most potent and useful foods given to man. So, what can we do? Humanity is stuck with this "safe" pasteurized milk in which the nutritional value has been altered and proteins denatured.

> From a nutritional standpoint, pasteurization is the equivalent of dropping an atomic bomb on your food. Whatever had been living in that food prior – delicate enzymes, probiotic bacteria, and various energetically-charged nutrients – is carpet-bombed with high heat and left for dead. It leaves in its wake a trail of compositional casualties like altered flavor and texture, denatured proteins, and lost vitamins and minerals ... among other damage.[48]

> Pasteurization is highly effective at killing things such as E-coli, salmonella, campylobacter, and listeria that can hang around in the gut and feces of even healthy cows. Raw milk, on the other hand, relies heavily on the skill of the farmer and the cleanliness of the operation to avoid contamination.[49]

Having been brought up on a farm with cows, I lost a great chance and opportunity of enjoying raw milk due to the fear of the above-mentioned diseases. The milk always had to be boiled first before use. Though I knew some people use it raw, this was considered a risky thing to do.

After learning the difference between pasteurized and raw milk, I decided to try raw milk, firstly raw cow's milk then raw goat's milk. I have now used the raw milk regularly for over 2 years, and I can confirm there is a big difference in taste. In fact, once you get accustomed to the raw milk, you can never again enjoy pasteurized milk, the flavors are miles apart. People use and enjoy pasteurized milk because they have no idea what the original taste of milk was. However, as mentioned above raw milk can cause sickness and diseases, so if you want to use raw milk *be sure* of the source. You have to know your suppliers. Raw milk is hard to find and more expensive, which makes it unattractive to people who are used to seeing so much cheap milk in the stores. I know many people are not able to get good raw organic milk; in fact, it is illegal in many countries to sell raw milk. My opinion on this was framed by Thomas Jefferson:

> If people let the government decide what foods they eat and what medicines they take, their bodies will soon be in as sorry a state as are the souls who live under tyranny.

One of the many benefits of raw milk may be its ability to promote the production of glutathione, which consists of three amino acids: cysteine, glycine, and glutamine. This is a powerful antioxidant that offers protection to cells from free radicals.

Raw milk provides the following:

- Fat-soluble vitamins A, D and K, K2 and E.
- Water-soluble vitamins such as vitamins C and B group vitamins.
- Short chain fatty acids, CLA (conjugated linoleic acid) whose many potential benefits include raising metabolic rate, helping to remove abdominal fat, boosting of muscle growth, reducing resistance to insulin, strengthening of the immune system, and lowering food allergy reactions.
- Essential minerals and electrolytes: calcium, magnesium, and potassium. zinc, iron, enzymes, and immunoglobulins IgG, IgA, IgM, IgE, IgD.

- Large, complex sugar/protein (glycoprotein) molecules (also known as antibodies) used by the immune system to find and deactivate pathogens such as bacteria and viruses.
- More than 60 digestive enzymes. These enzymes are destroyed during pasteurization, making pasteurized milk harder to digest. It also provides the body with Omega-3 fatty acids. Omega-3 fatty acids, though essential for human health, cannot be synthesized in the human body and must, therefore, be obtained from dietary sources. For vegetarians, raw milk from organic grass-fed animals is a good source of these fatty acids.
- Milk is a good source of protein such as whey and casein protein. Of these two types, whey protein is the most used especially in sports nutrition, but it's very heat sensitive meaning you will only be able to get the real whey from raw milk.
- Our bodies use amino acids as building blocks for protein. Nine are essential amino acids which we must get from food while the rest can be made through complex metabolic processes, these essential amino acids are histidine, isoleucine, leucine, lysine, methionine, phenylalanine, threonine, tryptophan, and valine. Raw cow's milk and indeed most other types of milk such as goat's milk have all 9 essential amino acids in varying amounts, and hence this makes raw milk a complete protein. Non-essential amino acids can be produced by the body, and these include serine, aspartic acid, beta alanine, glutamic acid, and others. Conditionally essential amino acids can be synthesized by the human body under certain circumstances; these include, ornithine, arginine, tyrosine, glycine, glutamine, cysteine, and proline. Apart from dairy and animal products, one can get amino acids from plants. One will need to combine certain foods in order to get complete protein such as combining grains with legumes or beans and being conscious of the food combination if your diet is entirely plant-based with no dairy or other animal products.
- Fats. Approximately two-thirds of the fat in milk is saturated. Saturated fat is really in a bad category due to its tendency to raise the bad cholesterol LDL. However, it appears saturated fats from raw milk may contribute to several vital roles in our bodies such as the construction of cell membranes and critical hormones to provide

energy storage and padding for delicate organs, as well as serving as a vehicle for essential fat-soluble vitamins.

- Carbohydrates. Lactose, or milk sugar, is the primary carbohydrate in cow's milk. People with lactose intolerance for one reason or another (age, genetics, etc.) no longer make the enzyme lactase and so can't digest milk. Fresh raw organically produced milk, with its lactose-digesting lactobacilli bacteria intact, may allow people with this intolerance to use milk and especially raw organic goat's milk. From my personal experience, I have noted that raw milk from goats doesn't cause lactose intolerance and this can be an alternative to people showing sensitivity to cow's milk. The other solution is taking lactase with your milk, and these will help in milk digestion.

Digestion Problems with Cow's Milk

Even after using raw organically produced milk, some people still complain of stomach problems, such as too much gas. Sometimes this happens with some milk and not others. Some research suggests that A2 casein from Jersey and Guernsey cows is easier to digest than A1. However, I will not go into details about this research. If one is still interested in using milk as one of their foods, it is important for them to find out, by trial and error, what foods agree or disagree with their stomach and digestive systems. I'm one of those who did a trial and error before deciding what to do. Being a vegetarian, I was not keen on dropping milk from my diet altogether because of the many nutritional benefits in the absence of other animal products. I wanted to benefit from all that the raw milk provides since it is also a complete protein with all 9 essential amino acids. I know I can still get this from plants, but it is more work since I must ensure I combine a few foods to ensure I get all the required amino acids.

However, I still experienced some gas unless I separated the whey and the casein. Not ready to give up on milk I decided to try raw goat's milk, and I was amazed at how calm my stomach was. I was stunned, and this made me research more on goat's milk. Though I liked the raw organic cow's milk, the taste, and availability, I gave in to raw goat's milk. Once again, I wondered why it took me many years to do this simple test to check which milk agrees with me. I had tried plant-derived milk, such as coconut, almond, and soya but I couldn't tolerate any of them.

Benefits of Goat's Milk

- Some research suggests that one of the main advantages of goat's milk is that it doesn't cause inflammation. This is due to the unique enzymatic make-up of goat's milk that soothes inflammation in the gut.
- Studies performed by the USDA and Prairie View A&M University link goat's milk to an increased ability to metabolize iron and copper.
- Goat's milk closely resembles human breast milk and contains A2 caseins which are much easier to digest and assimilate in the human body. Some cow's milk also has these A2 caseins.
- The fat molecules in goat's milk are much smaller than those found in cow's milk and hence easier to digest.
- Goat's milk has higher fatty acids percentage (35% in comparison to 17% in cow's milk) making it more nutritionally wholesome. By balancing our essential fatty acids in the body, we can reduce the chances of atherosclerosis, stroke, heart attack, and other coronary complications.
- Goat's milk is high in calcium, the amino acid tryptophan, and selenium, an essential trace mineral that supports the immune system.
- Goat's milk is a rich source of protein, which is an essential part of growth and development, as proteins are the building blocks of cells, tissue, muscle, and bone.
- People who are lactose intolerant may find goat's milk to be an excellent alternative source of milk. Goat's milk contains less lactose than cow's milk and passes through the digestive system more rapidly.
- Goat's milk, just like cow's milk, is a complete protein.
- The main disadvantage of raw goat's milk is its unavailability and cost.

Milk and Other Dairy Products

I mainly use milk only and homemade whey but avoid other dairy products such as cheese. I leave to the reader to decide on whether these milk products are right for them or not. Due to my tendency to have high-fat levels, I'm conscious of saturated fats, especially from a pasteurized source.

Though I still use raw milk and firmly believe that the original raw milk is good food for humans, I'm nevertheless concerned by the current milk production, the animal treatment, the use of hormones, antibiotics, pasteurization, and all that is happening in the commercial milk industry. I recently read the work of T. Colin Campbell, *The China Study*. Campbell appears to link consumption of animal protein with the development of cancer and heart disease, and he also argues that casein (a protein found in milk from mammals) is the most significant carcinogen we consume. This left me thinking about my belief that real milk was given as a food supplement to man. However, it is not stated what type of milk was used in the China study, whether raw or pasteurized and whether the milk was from A1 or A2 animals.

A1 casein protein is said to be very highly inflammatory for some people, and as we know, inflammation is the root of many diseases. This kind of inflammation can contribute to gastrointestinal issues like irritable bowel syndrome, Crohn's, leaky gut, colitis, autoimmune diseases, and skin problems like eczema and acne.

On the other hand, milk that contains mostly or exclusively A2 casein produces none of these inflammatory effects. Goat's milk contains only A2 casein, making it, protein-wise, the closest milk to human breast milk.[50]

Improving your health is a personal journey. Sometimes it is a trial and error journey because we are all different and what might appear good for one person is wrong for somebody else. In case you have not given up on milk, conduct your own research, look for organic farmers near where you live and start your own trial and error to see what works best for you.

What's the Solution?

Milk, just like other foods, such as wheat, potatoes, rice, and vegetables, was given to man as food. However, as we all know now, many people seem to be getting their health back once they stop taking dairy products. I believe most of the commercially produced milk today may be contributing to many of the problems associated with dairy foods. It's unfair to condemn the cow! It's the desire for profit and the high demand that has caused all these problems. If animals are fed with hormones, they are no longer feeding on just grass. Furthermore, when they are caged and no longer grazing freely, some will also be fed antibiotics, chemicals, and other stuff which is passed through the food chain thereby altering the purpose of the original natural milk. Then the already inferior product is heated to high temperatures whereby the remaining good is either destroyed or changed. It may sound alarming, but we end up with a "dead" substance which is why so many suppliers have to add back vitamins and other nutrients.

Finally, in view of what is happening to milk, I wonder if it would be safer to keep away from it altogether. I know this is not possible because it has its place in most people's daily diets. Milk production is a massive industry that contributes much to a country's economy. Having said that, it would be helpful if the farmers the world over could be helped to produce milk more responsibly. National governments should regulate milk production like they do other industries to ensure no antibiotics or hormones are passed to the public. More research needs to be done on the known effects of pasteurization and looking for better ways of making it safe without necessarily destroying the natural raw nutrients.

For me, the best solution would be to use raw organic milk from grass-fed animals that are not caged but are allowed to graze. These animals may be cows, goats or sheep. Goat's milk is easy to digest, and it's a good choice for people who can't tolerate cow's milk.

The other solution is to abstain from using milk and its products and use milk alternatives in the market. Perhaps, if one has space and time, one can become a farmer and produce their own milk. Keeping goats for milk production would be an excellent way to go if one has space and time.

It is worth noting that milk in its natural form is a superfood, but humans have changed it in all its stages, via genetic modification and cross-breeding, and through feeds, production, and processing. What we end up with is something inferior, but since it looks the same, we can't tell the difference. However, time has revealed that something is wrong as we have increased cases of milk intolerance and allergies.

Fresh raw milk from healthy well-fed animals is a living unprocessed whole food. Produced hygienically it poses no risk and has long been proven to aid many health problems such as eczema, asthma, and arthritis. Goat's milk is far more easily digested and absorbed than cow's milk and can be enjoyed by many people with lactose intolerance and allergy to cow's milk.

Raw milk is a living whole food that contains enzymes, a biodiversity of beneficial bacteria, sugars, proteins, fats, minerals, antibodies, and other essential elements needed to nourish a growing baby.

Raw milk also contains a complementary immune system that provides an environment that tends to suppress the growth of pathogenic bacteria in favor of beneficial lactic acid producing bacteria. Raw milk inside of the animal generally does not contain bacteria; however, as the milk exits the breast or teat canal, protective resident bacteria join the raw milk to complete its genome.[51]

Today milk has been condemned by some as food to be avoided if you want to be healthy. I agree—the pasteurized milk in the stores in its current form could be causing problems and should be used sparingly if at all.

Chapter 7: Meat

It is easier to talk about meat than milk because so many people are now abandoning the use of it as food. They have reached the conclusion that meat is not good for them. I'm happy to be writing about this at a time when many doctors, dieticians, and nutritionists agree on the non-use of meat, or at least its reduction. Dr. Ellsworth Wareham, who is 103 at the time I'm writing this book, has been a vegan for over half his life. In a place like Japan, some long-living citizens are not vegans, but their use of meat is very minimal. They also enjoy seafood (see M. Daisen's *Only in Japan*).[52]

Actually, for many poor people meat has always been a luxury. At one time in the UK and many other parts of the world, the poor would raise animals on their farms but sell them for meat. Killing their own animals for household consumption would be rare, though perhaps once in a while a chicken might be eaten, or maybe a goat/sheep if there was a special occasion.

However, not everyone is yet convinced that they should not eat meat. The people I have encountered rely on the teaching of Moses where he allowed the children of Israel to eat meat. What we fail to appreciate is, this was way after the flood. This was a permissive will rather than a perfect will. The food changed; the human body never did.

> It was said to them of old time, "Thou shalt not kill, for life is given to all by God and that which God has given let not man take away." For I tell you truly from one mother proceeds all that lives upon the Earth … and whoso eats the flesh of slain beasts, eats of the body of death … God commanded your forefathers thou shalt not kill, but their hearts were hardened, and they killed. Then Moses desired that at least they should not kill men and he suffered them to kill beasts. And then the heart of your forefathers was hardened yet more, and they killed men and beasts likewise. But I do say to you kill neither men, nor beast, nor yet the food which goes into your mouth. (*Essene Gospel of Peace Book 1*)[53]

> About noon the following day as they were on their journey and approaching the city, Peter went up on the roof to pray. He became hungry and wanted something to eat, and while the meal was being prepared, he fell into a trance. He saw heaven opened and something like a large sheet being let down to Earth by its four corners. It

contained all kinds of four-footed animals, as well as reptiles and birds. Then a voice told him, "Get up, Peter. Kill and eat." "Surely not, Lord!" Peter replied. "I have never eaten anything impure or unclean." The voice spoke to him a second time, "Do not call anything impure that God has made clean." (*Acts 10:9–15*)

Though some people may use the above scriptures in the Bible to say that killing of animals for food is okay, it is good to note that Peter's vision is God preparing Peter for something unusual for him to do, to mix with the Gentiles, who according to the Jews were unclean. The animals in this vision represent the non-Jews whom God had accepted and were no longer unclean. The passage, therefore, is not talking about meat-eating literally.

Some people also refer to the following message while discussing the issue of the food we eat, while they try to say it doesn't matter what you put in the mouth:

> "Not what goes into the mouth defiles a man; but what comes out of the mouth, this defiles a man." … Then Peter answered and said to Him, "Explain this parable to us." So, Jesus said, "Are you also still without understanding? Do you not yet understand that whatever enters the mouth goes into the stomach and is eliminated? But those things which proceed out of the mouth come from the heart, and they defile a man. For out of the heart proceed evil thoughts, murders, adulteries, fornications, thefts, false witness, blasphemies. These are *the things* which defile a man, but to eat with unwashed hands does not defile a man." (*Matthew 15:11, 15–20*)

As we can clearly see, the Pharisees had accused Jesus and the disciples of eating without washing their hands, and it is from this context that He gave this parable. The dirt from non-washing of hands cannot be compared with the issues that proceed from our hearts as mentioned.

Many researchers, doctors, and nutritionists such Dr. T. Colin Campbell and Dr. Caldwell Esselstyn (*Knives Over Forks*) are also showing the world that meat from animals can cause many diet-related diseases. Even in the beginning in Genesis 1:29, meat was not part of the diet of man, but this changed along the way in Genesis chapter 9.

Despite that, we know not everything that is lawful to eat is beneficial to our bodies. Though I'm gracious to all those who believe there is no need to change, I can't consciously go back to accept that killing of innocent animals for food is lawful. To me what now makes meat not to be part of my diet, is both its source (animal killing) as well as health reasons. Initially, it was for health reasons only. As 1 Corinthians 10:23 notes, "All things are lawful for me but not all things are helpful."

The apostle Paul asked for tolerance between meat eaters and vegetarians (Romans 14:1–2), when he wrote, "Accept the one whose faith is weak, without quarreling over disputable matters. One person's faith allows them to eat anything, but another, whose faith is weak, eats only vegetables." For me, 2000 years after those words were written, it appears the weaker brother was right after all. But judge for yourself and do what is right.

To the people in the Essene Gospel, Jesus kept quoting the law, "It was said of them of old," meaning He was citing the original legislation which appeared not to have been clearly understood.

> Thou shall not kill for life is given to all by God and that which God has given let no man take away. Kill not, neither eat the flesh of your innocent prey … but the flesh and the blood which quickens it shall ye not eat. He who eats the flesh of slain beasts eats of the body of death … and their death will become his death. (*Essene Gospel of Peace Book 1*)[54]

I was terrified and cried when I read these words. Since the day I read these writings concerning meat I have never knowingly tasted any. I was, however, sorry for myself because this truth was revealed to me later in my life after a lifetime of eating meat. I was guilty directly or indirectly. I was furious because I wondered why this information was never made available to me. I had spent about two years or more trying to stop eating meat because I didn't know whether that was good or not. So, when finally this "truth" was thrown in front of my face, that it could be morally wrong to kill animals for food, I felt sorry for my own participation in the killing of animals for food.

The killing of animals for food is an adapted method of feeding and not that which was designed initially. I realize we have enough food and therefore we do not need to kill animals for food anymore. Initially, my food shopping was meat based, and other foods were just additions. I believed in eating protein from animals and how on Earth could I survive without it?! God made provision for people long ago, and the land is always being renewed for man, there is still plenty for us to eat. Plant food is plentiful and delicious, available and in most cases requiring little or no cooking. Eating a plant-based, vegetarian or even a vegan diet requires thought and preparation if one is to get all the nutrients necessary. Yet once you get into the routine, it is the easiest way of eating.

When I first refrained from eating meat products, I experienced a time of body weakness and unwellness. After reading widely, I was able to introduce foods into my diet such as starches which I had previously avoided due to fear of weight gain. I also realized I must take enough fruits and vegetables for the body to be strong and healthy. From my experience, I would encourage anyone who wants to transition to get enough information and to have an idea of what foods they should eat. There is plenty of tasty plant-based food out there, but you must discover it for yourself if your change is going to be permanent.

I couldn't complain about what I was going through during my time of change, though I had a lot of opposition. I was searching for answers, and I asked God to reveal the truth to me, and it was dropped into my mind to seek what the Essenes ate. I had read in the book, *The Law of Light* by Lars Muhl[55] the idea that Jesus may have lived among the sect of Jews called the Essenes, and so did John the Baptist and Mari and Yoasaph (Mary and Joseph). In the time of my research and confusion, I wanted to know what kind of diet they followed, and whether Jesus had mentioned anything to do with meat. I had seen in some other writings that Jesus was a vegetarian, but I had not believed them. Really that was all I wanted to know, but I got more than I bargained for. It was not just whether one should eat meat or not but why it is wrong to kill animals for food. It was mind-blowing. It was a shock for me to know this information was there and it has been for many years.

It's is true that so many have no idea that Jesus ended the shedding of animal blood for sacrifice as well as for food.

> Is it not written in the prophets, put your blood sacrifices to your burnt offerings and way with them and cease ye from eating of flesh, for I spoke not your fathers nor commanded them when I brought them out of Egypt concerning these things? (*The Gospel of the Holy Twelve; also known as the Essenes New Testament*)[56]

> For I did not speak to your fathers, or command them in the day that I brought them out of the land of Egypt, concerning burnt offerings or sacrifices. But this is what I commanded them, saying, 'Obey My voice, and I will be your God, and you shall be My people. And walk in all the ways that I have commanded you, that it may be well with you.' Yet they did not obey or incline their ear, but followed the counsels and the dictates of their evil hearts, and went backward and not forward. (*Jeremiah 7:22–24*)

As a middle-aged man, Dr. Wareham spent a lot of time in the operating room cutting into one patient after another who had heart problems. There, he noticed something: patients who were vegetarian mostly had much cleaner and smoother arteries than those who ate meat. The arteries of meat-eaters tended to be full of calcium and plaque. So, he made a choice. He decided to become a vegan. Dr. E. Wareham is now 103 by the time I am writing this book. He asked this question, "If you can live a long happy life without harming others why wouldn't you." I believe he meant without harming animals.

I noticed that some long-living Christians are Seventh-day Adventists, and I wondered what the connection was. When it comes to lifestyle, Seventh-day Adventists believe the human body is the temple of God and thus should be cared for properly. Because of this, many Adventists abstain from harmful substances like alcohol and tobacco and maintain a vegetarian diet.

Ultimately our lives are in the hands of our maker. He already knows our lifespan and therefore seeking him through prayer and meditation will ensure we get the necessary help as we journey towards eternity. It is not only a long life that people want but also lives with fewer problems such as diseases. I believe in the near future there will be a significant distinction between those who follow the original laws and those who support the permitted laws. In all this, the idea is to try to follow that which is beneficial for us.

When to Eat our Meals

> Eat only when the sun is highest in the heavens, and again when it is set. And you will **never see disease**, for such finds favor in the eyes of the Lord. And if you will that the angels of God rejoice in your body, and that Satan shun you afar, then sit but once in the day at the table of God. And then your days **will be long** upon the Earth, for

this is pleasing in the eyes of the Lord. (*Essene Gospel of Peace Book 1*)[57]

Though there is a strong belief that one should not miss breakfast, stating that breakfast is king, this does not entirely agree with the above statement. Where I grew up, we never used to eat in the morning. We only used to take a cup of milky tea or milk. This would last us until lunchtime and sometimes up to dinner. We thought it was shameful to eat in the morning, that it would give us stomach upsets. I wonder why it was like that? It is as if by instinct our parents knew something. However, this way of living was dropped when we went to the city and saw how other people were living. We thought our ideas were inferior and quickly adopted new ways. I was quite upset when I realized my mother was right after all; she never gave us a substantial breakfast in the morning because it would cause us stomach indigestion, but we didn't follow this through but got into the new ways, and heavy breakfasts were introduced regardless of the amount of dinner one took previously, and this was followed by lunches and snacks in between. As Arnold Ehret said, "Life is a tragedy of nutrition."[58] Not only the amount and content but also the timing of it.

I know there is a lot of scientific evidence to support breakfast. The word breakfast is two words joined together to mean "breaking the fast." This, I believe, can be done at any time, not necessarily in the morning. It can be done after 11am and still be breakfast. The above statement of eating when the sun is up is a form of intermittent fasting which I have discussed elsewhere. There is growing evidence that intermittent fasting (a fast of 16–18 hours) helps in weight loss and other metabolic issues. The benefits of this method of eating mimic the ones of full fasting. The idea is that you allow the body to use the stored glycogen and fats before you introduce new foods.[59]

It is not easy to do away with the morning breakfast, especially if one is accustomed to having one. Aiming for quality instead of quantity is very important. Instead of eating a heavy breakfast one can start with a light one of fruits or fresh homemade vegetable/fruit juice or your usual cup of tea. However, some people take their breakfast in the morning and avoid the lunch break. The choice depends on one's working schedule, and the time they eat their dinner. The idea is to have several hours between your last meal and your next one.

In his book, *Mucusless Diet Healing System*, Professor Arnold Ehret stated that hundreds of severe cases were cured by the non-breakfast-fast but cautioned that people would experience some headaches if breakfast was eliminated for the first one or two days. Afterward, however, one feels much better, works better and enjoys luncheon better than ever.

It has been my experience too, whenever I don't take breakfast, that I enjoy my lunch and the food tastes delicious. I'm more alert, and this definitely assists me in the area of calorie restriction.

As written in the *Essene Gospel of Peace Book 1*, Jesus took this further and recommended that those who can do so should have only one meal a day. Whoa! That is a real stretch! However, several people are doing this programme all over the world and are claiming a lot of health benefits. The spiritual pledge of this plan is *that Satan will shun you afar, and your days will be long on Earth.* The promise itself is enticing, but I know that sometimes the heart is willing, but the body is weak. With God's help, this is possible. One just needs to ensure their one daily meal is packed up with enough nutrients to keep them healthy, and so it must be nutrient-dense. The one meal per day plan should consist of the recommended foods to ensure the body is getting enough nutrients and energy to keep it going. It's another form of intermittent fasting. The hours between meals are what makes this a perfect kind of intermittent fasting.

I also know due to work and other arrangements, it may also not be possible to eat during the day and hence eating in the morning makes sense. I have taken breakfast for many years during my adult life, but this truth was never available to me, but now it is very beneficial to our bodies.

Please note the above is an ideal suggestion. There are those who prefer to take breakfast and miss lunch while there are those who miss dinners and have breakfast. I have only laid down here what was suggested in those early days, and though it may appear difficult in the beginning, it's worth trying.

Disclaimer, this is not medical advice and is not for young children, pregnant women and for those on medication. Please follow your doctor's advice.

How we Should Take our Meals

We are generally programmed to eat at certain times of the day. However, your body may not be ready to eat at meal times; either you don't feel hungry because you are full or unwell, or there are things on your mind that have caused you to lose your appetite. In such circumstances, it is advisable not to feed the body until the time when you are ready to eat. In the *Essene Gospel of Peace Book 1*, Jesus taught the people who asked for his help to only eat when hungry, only when summoned by the angel of appetite.

Around 10–20 minutes before having our meals it is a good idea to take a glass of water. This prepares the digestive system for the incoming hard work of digestion. The water will help clean up the system ready for the new food. Ideally, no liquids should be taken together with the food. While eating we should get into the habit of breathing long and deep during our meals while chewing our food properly. Breathing deeply helps us support the body with more oxygen and helps to get things moving in the digestive system. Chewing food properly helps it to get liquidized, and this enables more absorption, making digestion less strenuous for our digestive system. As our mothers used to say, eat slowly and chew your food. Dr. Michael Klaper once said, "We are what we absorb," and not necessarily what we eat.[60]

Chewing our food correctly and liquidizing it in the mouth before it goes to the stomach increases nutrient absorption, and this habit needs to be practiced. Therefore, eating slowly is advisable. This is a practice worth trying.

In mindful eating, we are encouraged to eat slowly, to appreciate the food fully in smell, texture, and taste. This practice will enable us to eat more slowly naturally, and this will be followed by a sense of fullness which will lead us to eat less. This can also help weight loss if done consistently.

Being mindful when we are eating food allows the body to respond appropriately to what it's doing. If you eat whilst worrying about your next meeting, the body is in stress mode, and digestion is compromised. Eating mindfully also allows for the proper signals to be sent to the brain when we're full, preventing us overeating.[61]

Most of our daily food intake should be raw or mildly cooked. This is a very challenging statement, but it should be the goal of every optimum-health seeker. There is a strong belief that cooking releases some nutrients from food. While this may be the case, it only releases some nutrients after it has destroyed others. Most vitamins get destroyed or are reduced by heat, while most proteins are also denatured. We have become so accustomed to eating cooked and hot food that it is hard to imagine life without cooked food.

Seasonal Eating

> Eat always when the table of God is served before you and eat always of that which you find upon the table of God. For I tell you truly, God knows well what your body needs, and when it needs. (*Essene Gospel of Peace Book 1*)[62]

The above statement means that we should eat food that the earth is producing wherever we live. People all over the world have different fruits and vegetables that come at different seasons. God in His wisdom knows what is good at every season. Eating the fruits growing on our trees and what the earth is producing at different seasons is probably the way to go. Growing up on a farm away from the city, we enjoyed seasonal fruits and crops. However, when we moved to the city, it was a different story. Today, however, due to globalization, we can eat the same food all year round imported from different parts of the world. London is never short of any kind of food, and so it is difficult to observe seasonal eating.[63] It's not clear what the eventual effect of this will be for our bodies. Our bodies require different nutrition as the seasons change. The foods we eat in winter should be different from what we eat in summer. But if we do not grow our own vegetables in a garden, it is not easy to know what is in season, especially if one relies on a supermarket for shopping. This contributes too to our inability to know exactly what the earth is producing at any particular time.

Weekly Fasting

In the *Essene Gospel of Peace Book 1* , it is recorded that eating for 6 days and fasting on the 7th day is ideal for spiritual and physical maintenance. This was mainly for spiritual development, as they never used to work on the Sabbath day—the day of the fast—but would spend the day seeking spirituality.

> And let not food trouble the work of the angels in your body throughout the seventh day. (*Essene Gospel of Peace Book 1*)

Currently, we have proponents of 5:2 diet which is a form of intermittent fasting which mimics the above statement as an eating idea. Here people eat for 5 days and then fast or reduce their calorie intake to 500–600 calories for 2 days.

Doctor and journalist Michael Mosley presented the diet as "genuinely revolutionary" and published *The Fast Diet* book in January 2013, while Kate

Harrison released her version titled, *The 5:2 Diet Book*. This diet is popular with many people because it does not have any food restriction during the 5-day window of eating.

> The greatest discovery by modern man is the power to rejuvenate himself physically, mentally, and spiritually with rational fasting. (Dr. Paul C. Bragg, *The Miracle of Fasting*)[64]

Food Portions

> And when you eat, never eat unto fullness. (*Essene Gospel of Peace Book 1*)[65]

> A full stomach does not like to think. (*Old German Proverb*)[66]

If we stick to the recommended food table, it will be difficult to overeat. The most important thing is to ensure that one eats good energetic foods that will supply our bodies with daily energy, enough nutrients to maintain all the systems of the body (aim at quality, not quantity). When our daily feast is composed of fruits, vegetables, grains, nuts, honey, and raw milk (if one takes milk) we are bound to be on the right track. All these should be eaten in moderation and the right portions.

> Would thou enjoy a long life, a healthy body, and a vigorous mind and be acquainted also with the wonderful works of God, labor in the first place to bring thy appetite to reason? (*Benjamin Franklin*)[67]

Do not eat often, not more than twice in a day. I know most of us eat more than twice or even three times a day. Eating many times a day is counterproductive to our body's constitution; eating in moderation as far as quantity, timing, and content are concerned is excellent for our bodies to enable them to carry the work of digestion, elimination, and healing. With proper planning and determination, we can ensure that we are getting enough nutrients at planned mealtimes without eating all the time. When I learned about the difference this kind of eating makes, I started to see a lot of difference in my life. I especially began to lose weight without the struggles I had previously experienced.

Drinking and Smoking

Though many people in the world, including Christians, drink alcohol, there is an interesting quote in the book of Essenes that talks about drinking:

> And take no delight in any drink, nor in any smoke from Satan, waking you by night and making you sleep by day. For I tell you truly, all the drinks and smokes are an abomination in the eyes of God. (*Essene Gospel of Peace Book 1*)[68]

I leave that as food for your thoughts and your choice.

Chapter 8: Exercise

Physical exercise is any bodily activity that enhances or maintains physical fitness and overall health and wellness. It helps in regulating digestive health, building and maintaining healthy bone density, muscle strength, and joint mobility among many benefits that are derived from physical activity.

> Those who think they have no time for bodily exercise will sooner or later have to find time for illness. (*Edward Stanley, Earl of Derby, 1826–93*)

> Follow the example of the running water, the wind as it blows, the rising and setting of the sun, the growing plants and trees, the beasts as they run and gambol, the wane and waxing of the moon, the stars as they come and go again; all these do move and do perform their labors. For all which has life does move, and only that which is dead is still. (*Essene Gospel of Peace Book 1*)[69]

For the majority of people, the way we live today is very different from the times when people worked every day on farmland. In those days, it would have been strange for somebody to sit down for the whole day; this would only happen if they were unwell. Today, most work involves sitting on a chair at a desk in front of a computer for the whole day at least 5 days a week for most weeks of the year. This change in working lifestyle has come at a cost and has contributed to the sedentary lifestyle of our generation. It is not by choice that people must work that way. Despite all of these challenges we are supposed to create time and ensure we are moving our bodies for health reasons. Because of the nature of our work the current regime of vigorous exercise and gym going has come into play. Signing up to a sports center gave me the discipline and commitment to do more exercise. If one is unable to be consistent in one's method of exercise, such as walking, one can probably apply different approaches. One can join a dancing group, go swimming, walk up and down the stairs and so on. All this will require conscious thought and effort, but when one remembers the benefits, one is helped to follow through.

For exercise to give us further benefits such as healing and physical fitness, we must make our movement more intense and longer lasting. As mentioned above, the need to remind people to exercise has been necessitated by our lifestyle because in the olden days people worked in the farm from morning till evening and hence there was no need for further exhaustion of the body. Regardless of the nature of our work we need to create time for movement.

> Walking is man's best medicine. If you are in a bad mood go for a walk. If you are still in a bad mood go for another walk. (*Hippocrates*)[70]

> All parts of the body which have a function, if used in moderation and exercised in labors in which each is accustomed, become thereby healthy, well developed and age more slowly, but if unused they become liable to disease, defective in growth and age quickly. (*Hippocrates*)[71]

Although exercising can be challenging to start with, the benefits are worth it. Just doing a small amount of exercise per day can give you the inspiration to keep improving. In addition to reducing excess fat, exercise can tone muscle, help you overcome or reduce numerous health problems, improve energy and mood as well as promote more restful sleep. Just walking in natural surroundings can help the body and mind rejuvenate. Remember always:

> That which is used develops. That which is not used wastes away. (*Hippocrates*)[72]

> Exercise is a journey, not a destination. It must be continued for the rest of your life. We do not stop exercising because we grow old—we grow old because we stop exercising. (*Kenneth Cooper*)[73]

> Physical fitness is not only one of the most important keys to a healthy body; it is the basis of dynamic and creative intellectual activity. (*John F. Kennedy*)[74]

A study conducted in Denmark suggested that people who are active for at least three hours per week had a 40% lower risk of dying prematurely than people who were less active.

The UK government recommends that people should do at least 150 minutes of moderate aerobic activity, such as cycling or brisk walking, every week. This should include strength exercises on two or more days in a week that work all the major muscles in the legs, hips, back, abdomen, chest, shoulders, and arms.

The following is an Australian government recommendation on physical activity which also gives us good advice:

- Doing any physical activity is better than doing none. If you currently do no physical activity, start by doing some, and gradually build up to the recommended amount.
- Be active on most, preferably all, days every week.
- Accumulate 150 to 300 minutes (2 ½ to 5 hours) of moderate intensity physical activity or 75 to 150 minutes (1 ¼ to 2 ½ hours) of vigorous intensity physical activity, or an equivalent combination of both moderate and vigorous activities, each week.
- Do muscle-strengthening activities on at least 2 days each week.

The following also is a recommendation for older Australians.

- Older people should do some form of physical activity, no matter what their age, weight, health problems or abilities.
- Older people should be active every day in as many ways as possible, doing a range of physical activities that incorporate fitness, strength, balance, and flexibility.
- Older people should accumulate at least 30 minutes of moderate intensity physical activity on most, preferably all, days.
- Older people who have stopped physical activity, or who are starting a new physical activity, should begin at a level that is easily manageable and gradually build up the recommended amount, type, and frequency of activity.
- Older people who continue to enjoy a lifetime of vigorous physical activity should carry on doing so in a manner suited to their capability into later life, provided recommended safety procedures and guidelines are adhered to.

Exercising regularly can keep your heart and arteries young: "The secret to youthful looks and a long life could be working out five times a week, reveals study." The study states the following conclusions:

- Arteries stiffen as people grow older, but exercise could keep them young. Arteries are the main blood vessels which supply blood to the body. They are elastic tubes but tend to become stiffer as people get older.

- People should exercise four or more times per week to protect the main arteries; more exercise is needed to benefit all areas. All arteries, including the larger ones which supply blood to the chest and abdomen, are healthier among people who exercise four or more times per week.
- Exercising less is still beneficial but does not maintain all blood vessels.

A further study from Johns Hopkins University in Baltimore, in May 2018 stated the following:

- Going for a walk or a bike ride for the recommended two-and-a-half hours a week can reduce the risk of chronic illness in just six years.
- Failing to do any exercise or stopping after leading a previously active life can increase the chance of getting a devastating condition.
- Those who progress from no exercise to consistently doing the recommended amount within six years cut their risk by nearly a quarter.[75]

Jack Lalanne (1914–2011) who was an American fitness, exercise, and nutrition expert, used to say, *"Exercise is King, and Nutrition is Queen, and together you have a kingdom."*[76] He was active throughout his life and passed due to a pneumonia attack. He was an excellent example of what exercise can do to help us achieve better health.

Ernestine Shepperd, who at 82 years old is the world's oldest female bodybuilder, reminded me that it does not matter how old one is, with determination and consistency one can still make a lot of difference in their lives and body if they incorporate exercise as one of the ways to improve their lifestyle. She started to work out aged 56, and 26 years on, she is still strong.

Chapter 9: New Lifestyle

Depending on where you are in your journey of health, this book will help you get started with a new way of living. It took many years for you to reach where you are, and it will take a while for you to restore your health completely. However, once you get started, you will begin to experience small positive changes which will lead you to more success. The initial positive changes that you see will energize you to continue the journey. To be restored to health or to the desired weight, we must be willing to analyze our lives and see where we have left the best, original path. Some may not feel the need to do so because they are still in good health. However, it is still a good idea to make some changes. Some people are already suffering health problems caused or exacerbated by bad diet and unhealthy lifestyle. In order to overcome diet and lifestyle problems, one must be willing to change. This is a personal journey and will require personal sacrifice and determination. Once you decide you want to change, you have to be ready to see it through despite opposition. Discard old habits. All those things that have brought you problems, or can cause trouble in the future, need to be abandoned; you do not need them. It's not a simple process, and it requires determination and inner strength and a great desire to be different. However, change can only start from within somebody and must involve the mind and the heart before it is eventually expressed in your actions and your body. Without a sincere desire within, the changes you make will only last for a while, and you will eventually slip back to your old life. Deep within human nature, there seem to be forces that lead us to do the wrong things.

> Beelzebub the prince of devils the source of every evil lies in the body of all the sons of men. He is death the lord of every plaque. (*Essene Gospel of Peace Book 1*)[77]

In the Essene Gospel, Jesus alerted the sick of the possibility of these contrary spirits that can lie hidden within the bodies of human beings that would cause them trouble.

The journey to health does not involve diet alone, but a more profound confrontation with these powers that chain us to misery. They tempt us at our weakest points with the aim of destroying our wholeness. Food is one method that these evil powers use as they entice us to overeat and to eat the wrong things. The result of such living is that our bodies become ill and we spend the rest of our lives fighting sickness. These powers, if they are not causing us to overeat, are filling our thoughts and feelings with bitterness, sorrow, regret, fear, envy, greed, jealousy, trauma, unforgiveness, etc. All these things make us sick mentally and prevent us from living as we were meant to. Therefore, for any meaningful change to take place, prayer and meditation—as well as a change of diet and lifestyle—must take place. It is a process, and with the help of God our Father, change is possible.

The Importance of Keeping Our Mind and Heart Clean

The following Bible verse derived from Proverbs 4:23 helps us to really understand how important our heart is. I have shown different versions to help us get the meaning. Our thoughts/feelings really run our lives whether they be good or bad.

> Keep your heart with all diligence, for out of it spring the issues of life. (*NKJV*)

> Above everything else, guard your heart; for it is the source of life's consequences. (*CJB*)

> Above all else, guard your heart, for everything you do flows from it. (*NIV*)

> Keep vigilant watch over your heart; that's where life starts. (*The Message*)

This verse is a gem among others. I never knew the effect of my dwelling on things such as sorrow or fear would so affect my thinking and feelings and hence shape my lifestyle. These negative issues of life eventually cause our soul to lose energy, which in turn affects the wellbeing of our physical body. We need to be aware of the need to endeavor to always keep our minds fixed on beautiful things and beautiful feelings.

It is said that all thoughts taking form in the brain descend into the pituitary gland via the hypothalamus and the negativity and emotional trauma they contain is passed on to the organs, blood, and the entire body causing a depletion in energy and eventual illness.

Before the "new you" can come along, you must abandon some old ways; you can't build on old habits and old ways of doing things. You cannot put new wine into old wineskins.

The sick and desperate Essenes were carefully advised to diligently take a 7-day fast (which we can call a detox stage) if they were going to restore their health completely. It was fitting that they go through this demanding stage first because that was the only way they could get rid of all the bad things in their bodies. This way they were to be delivered from the clutches of Satan, through prayer, good thoughts, by use of water, air, and sunlight and by embracing loving thoughts and peace. They were to do this even before they were advised on what to eat. Later Jesus taught them about the right kind of nutrition. This needed to be done urgently. Otherwise, they would go back to what they used to do, and the same old problems would return.

Remember, whenever Jesus healed the sick, he told them to go and sin no more. It is the same today. If our bodies are healed by whatever method, we need to ask some questions about why we got sick in the first place. Some people think this is not a valid question, but some diseases are diet and lifestyle related and hence changes in these areas must take place; otherwise, it is possible to relapse into ill-health. Due to lack of awareness or knowledge many people do not know how to keep their healing, for they soon go back and do those things they did before they got sick.

7-Day Fast

They say 7 is a perfect number! Though the reason for the 7-day fast may not be fully understood, nevertheless the sick among the Essenes were told to fast for 7 days:

> But wait penitently for the seventh day which is sanctified by God. Renew yourselves and fast. For I tell you truly that Satan and his plagues may only be cast out by fasting and by prayer ... except you fast, you shall never be freed from the power of Satan and from all diseases that come from Satan. (*Essene Gospel of Peace Book 1*)[78]

As we have seen before there are many benefits of fasting and taking a few days of fasting will be very beneficial if you want to kick start your new lifestyle. For more details on fasting, please read earlier chapter on fasting.

Benefits of Drinking Water

Drinking Water Helps Maintain the Balance of Body Fluids. The functions of these bodily fluids include digestion, absorption, circulation, the creation of saliva, transportation of nutrients, and maintenance of body temperature. Since our body is made of 60% water, we need to ensure we are getting enough to allow the body to function efficiently.

Water Increases Brain Power and Provides Energy. Adequate fluids and electrolytes help the body muscle cells to work well, and lack of enough bodily fluids can make their performance suffer.

Water Promotes Healthy Weight Management and Weight Loss. "If one chooses water or a non-caloric beverage over a caloric beverage and/or eat a diet higher in water-rich foods that are healthier and more filling."[79]

Water Helps Flush Out Toxins. Kidneys do an amazing job of cleansing and ridding our body of toxins as long as your intake of fluids is adequate. Scientists say the main toxin in the body is blood urea nitrogen. One may develop kidney stones if there is no sufficient water intake.

Water Helps Improves Complexion. "The skin contains plenty of water and functions as a protective barrier to prevent excess fluid loss. Dehydration makes the skin look drier and more wrinkled which can be improved with proper hydration," says Atlanta dermatologist Kenneth Ellner, "But once you are adequately hydrated, the kidneys take over and excrete excess fluids."[80]

Water Helps Maintain Normal Bowel Function. When you don't get enough fluid, the colon pulls water from stools to maintain hydration, and the result is constipation. Taking sufficient and enough fiber ensures the bowels are functioning well.

Water Helps Regulate Your Body Temperature. Drinking fluids and especially water helps to ensure the body temperature remains at optimum levels.

Benefits of Deep Breathing

This kind of breathing is also known as diaphragmatic breathing, abdominal breathing, belly breathing, and paced respiration. Deep abdominal breathing encourages full oxygen exchange; that is, the beneficial trade of incoming oxygen for outgoing carbon dioxide. Not surprisingly, this type of breathing slows the heartbeat and can lower or stabilize blood pressure.[81]

The same research states that shallow breathing limits the diaphragm's range of motion, which causes the lowest part of the lungs not to get a full share of oxygenated air which can make one feel short of breath.

Carbon dioxide is a natural waste product of our body's metabolism. The benefits of breathing deeply help the systems in the body to process this more efficiently.

The following also are other benefits of deep breathing as noted by many different sources and *Conscious Lifestyle*.[82]

1. Breath Increases Energy. Oxygen is an essential natural resource required by our cells, and though we can stay without food and even water for some time, we cannot survive for many minutes without breathing.

2. Breath Improves the Respiratory System. It helps us to release tension in the diaphragm and primary breathing muscles, relieving many long-term respiratory issues such as asthma and breathlessness.

3. Breath Calms the Nervous System. Deep breathing activates the parasympathetic nervous system, bringing us into a relaxed state.

4. Breath Strengthens the Lymphatic System. Deep breathing can play an essential role in protecting the body from bacteria, viruses, and other threats to our health.

5. Breath Releases Muscle Tension. Deep breathing helps to release us from uncomfortable feelings such as anger or pain.

6. Breath Improves the Cardiovascular System. Deep diaphragmatic breathing tones, massages, and increases circulation to the heart, liver, brain, and reproductive organs.

7. Breath Elevates the Digestive System. The benefits of deeper breathing include increased blood flow in the digestive tract, which encourages intestinal action and improves overall digestion.

8. Breath Affects Our Mental State. The quality of our breath helps to relax the mind and enhance the ability to learn, focus, concentrate, and memorize.

In summary, the many benefits of deep breathing include a reduction in stress and blood pressure, strengthening of abdominal and intestinal muscles, and relief of general body aches and pains. Deep breathing also promotes better blood flow, releases toxins from the body, and aids in healthy sleep. These benefits result in increased energy levels. Deep breathing releases endorphins throughout the body—the feel-good, natural painkillers created by our own bodies. We need to breathe long, deep, and often to get all the benefits.

Sunlight

While fasting, it is vital to ensure one goes out to get the sunlight. This may not be possible always for people living in cold areas where the sun is rare. However, it is good to fast in times when one can go outside, to get some sunlight. There are many benefits of exposing ourselves to the sunshine whenever possible for a considerable amount of time.

In a study conducted at the University of California, San Diego, researchers combined data from other surveys of satellite measurements of sunlight and cloud during the winter from 15 countries to estimate the serum level of vitamin D metabolite of people living in 177 countries. The compilation of data revealed a link between low vitamin D levels and the risk of colorectal and breast cancer. According to the researchers, raising the serum levels was found to be ideal for cancer prevention, which means 600,000 cases of breast and colorectal cancer could be prevented each year with sufficient exposure to sunlight. Dr. Cedric Garland of UC San Diego School of Medicine and Moores Cancer Center, the co-author of the study, said, "This could be best achieved with a combination of diet, supplements and short intervals—10 or 15 minutes a day in the sun."[83]

Benefits of Sunlight

Sufficient Supply of Vitamin D. The most important advantage of exposure to sunlight is its ability to boost your body's vitamin D supply. The National Institutes of Health says at least 1,000 different genes that control every tissue in the body are linked to being regulated by vitamin D3 which is produced by the skin's response to UV radiation during sun exposure.[84]

Vitamin D helps regulate the amount of calcium and phosphate in the body. These nutrients are useful in keeping our bones, teeth, and muscles healthy.

A deficiency in these vitamins can lead to rickets in children and osteomalacia in adults.[85]

Enhances Your Mood. Regular sunlight exposure can naturally increase the serotonin levels in your body, making you more active and alert. In an article published by the National Institutes of Health (NIH), exposure to bright light is seen as an approach to increase serotonin without the use of drugs.[86]

Lowers Blood Pressure. Skin that is exposed to ultraviolet (UV) rays release a compound, nitric oxide, that reduces blood pressure.[87] In a recent study conducted at Edinburgh University, dermatologists studied the blood pressure of 34 volunteers under UV and heat lamps. The results of the study showed a significant drop in blood pressure after exposure to UV rays for an hour.

Protects from Melanoma. The skin's exposure to ultraviolet radiation of short wavelengths (UVB) has been linked to a decreased risk of melanoma in outdoor workers compared to their indoor counterparts, which suggests chronic sunlight exposure can have a protective effect.[88]

Although excessive sun exposure is an established risk factor for cutaneous malignant melanoma, continued high sun exposure was linked with increased survival rates in patients with early-stage melanoma.[89]

Prayer and Meditation

Fasting is also a time of prayer and meditation. As you renew your body, you will need to renew your thoughts and feelings. It is a time to ask for help from God to abandon all the negative thoughts and feelings while praying for the ability to embrace thoughts of love towards God and other human beings. Fasting can help one move towards this goal of the unconditional love of God. God loves us unconditionally and expects us to love unconditionally too. Without this achievement, it's difficult for our soul to be fully relieved of all the burdens and troubles of the ego. Unconditional love helps us reach the serenity status where the peace and joy of the Lord dwells and indeed where all things are possible because love is eternal and is stronger than death.

The Apostle Paul had a revelation when he wrote:

> Love is patient, love is kind. It does not envy, it does not boast, it is not proud. It does not dishonor others, it is not self-seeking, it is not

easily angered, it keeps no record of wrongs. Love does not delight in evil but rejoices with the truth. It always protects, always trusts, always hopes, always perseveres. (1 Corinthians 13:4)

After going through the cleansing stage, and having persisted for 7 days, it is important to start feeding your body with live foods. We eat live food when we eat foods in their natural form before they are either cooked, processed or destroyed by heat. However, the majority of the food that most people eat is cooked or processed. Both cooked and processed foods are tasty and delicious, sometimes with artificial additives to make them more appetizing. However, what most people are not aware of is that these processed foods have fewer nutrients and hence do not fully nourish our organs. The vitamins and other nutrients in them are either destroyed, reduced in their functions, or denatured.

Chapter 10: Supplementation

The practice of taking supplements is a very controversial one. There are those who say it's a waste of money and may pose some health risks. On the other hand, there are those who believe that supplements—if taken carefully and when needed—are essential in restoring and supporting healthy living.

Why People Take Supplements

Inability and failure to consume enough portions of fruit and vegetables consistently on a daily basis is part of the reason why supplements became a necessity. Most people eat cooked or processed foods and rarely eat enough raw fruit and vegetables. Since the nutrients received from cooked foods are denatured and reduced in value, using this kind of nutrient-deficient food for a long time will eventually lead to deficiencies that will require urgent attention such as supplementation. Such a person will need to improve on their diet so that they can naturally nourish their bodies. However, in the short term and as a crutch, supplementation may be required to support the body until the right levels are reached. People are typically given supplements of vitamins such as D when levels are too low. Vegans and vegetarians may sometimes need the additional support of vitamin B12 when their levels are low. Sometimes it is not possible to know what you are deficient in, and that is why people take multivitamins, multi-minerals and B complex among others. Due to the overuse of the soil and the use of chemicals, most home-grown foods contain fewer vitamins and minerals. As we have seen in the earlier chapters, the majority of the milk we use is pasteurized and has most of the vitamins, minerals, and proteins reduced, destroyed, or denatured, and hence people may still end up with deficiencies though eating what they consider to be a "healthy diet."

Having said that, if we load ourselves with enough fruit and vegetables in their raw form, and with organically produced raw milk from grass-fed animals, we will most likely be supporting our bodies with all the essential nutrients that they need, and so we will have no need for supplementation.

Generally, supplements are supposed to be used as a support as you heal yourself through proper nutrition and lifestyle change. Getting vitamins, minerals, amino acids from food is far better than getting extracted isolated vitamins or minerals. However, since the concentration in the foods we eat may not be sufficient to help in time of deficiencies, it's a good idea to support the body with supplements in the short term. However, they should not be used as a replacement for a good diet and should not be used for a long time. Ideally one should only use them if blood tests confirm that there is a deficiency. The best way to increase your levels is through foods such as fruits and vegetables and raw organically produced milk from grass-fed animals for milk users and try to get plenty of sunshine

In summary, the following are some of the reasons why some people may need supplements:

- Soil: the condition of the ground where the crops grow matters.
- Storage & transportation: Nutrients are destroyed, reduced during storage and transportation.
- Food portions: Eating less than the required portion of fruits and vegetables.
- Pasteurization: This method denatures, diminish, and destroys nutrients in food.
- Cooking of food: Just like pasteurization, most cooking also destroys and reduces the food's nutritional value.
- Food processing: Processing food also reduces its natural value.
- Lack of enough sunshine exposure: The sun not only provides vitamin D but many other benefits, some of which are unrecorded. Many studies have shown vitamin D shortage to be a root cause of many diseases.

Advantages of Taking Supplements

- Act as a crutch.
- Easily available.
- Easy to reach the bloodstream since they are micronutrients.
- Measurable especially during a time of deficiency.
- Controllable and easier to manage.
- Peace of mind especially when the deficiency has been reported—not sure whether the food you are eating will get you there, but supplements will bridge the gap as you try to build up the required nutrients from food.

Disadvantages of Taking Supplements

- Expensive.
- Limited only to the specific supplement you are taking, unlike with food where you get other nutrients as well, foods such as fruit, vegetables, and even milk come loaded with various vitamins and minerals.
- Risk of toxicity. It is very easy to exceed the limits with some vitamins, and this can cause toxicity. Most fat-soluble vitamins such as A, D, E, and K are fat-soluble and can cause toxicity if taken in excess because they can be stored in the body's fatty tissues. Water-soluble vitamins such as C and B complex do not cause toxicity because they dissolve in water and are not stored in the body.
- The use of many different supplements can be overwhelming on the liver.
- Very many contradicting reports on the safety and usefulness of supplements are causing a lot of confusion.

In my research, I have come across stories of many healthy people who take no supplements except vitamins B12 (especially vegans and vegetarians). There are others who take supplements such as vitamin D3 and claim a lot of benefits.

I think the way to supplementation is very personal and requires individual research. It is wrong to load your system with many vitamins and minerals for the sake of it when there is no need to. Some people assume the need even before they establish it through blood investigation. Depending on your circumstances, be proactive and ask your doctors for a blood test to check on the essential vitamins and minerals among other requirements. The results will give you an indication on whether you need to take supplements or not and if required, what quantity. Your body also may provide evidence of when it is suffering from a lack of vitamins and minerals, though it is difficult to know what area needs attention. Going for natural vitamins instead of synthetic ones is a good way to go. Always be careful about your liver and other organs as you load your body with medication and supplements.

Personally, I have used supplements to help restore my health. I was feeling poorly with lots of health problems, such as lack of energy, hair loss, a thyroid nodule, acid reflux, arthritis, etc. I was found to be deficient in vitamin D, and hence I had to take supplements. For some time, I took various supplements which I believe helped me as I built up my reserves through diet. I cannot categorically say that the supplements were wholly responsible for my health restoration because diet and lifestyle choices were involved as well. Since I live in a cold country, I regularly take Vitamins D3 and K2 to ensure I don't drop to the red zone again. I would also have loved to be taking vitamins C supplements, but my stomach is sensitive to direct vitamins C intake, so I can only get vitamin C from some food and vegetables in low form.

Chapter 11: Raw Plant-Based Diet

What is Plant-Based Nutrition?

A plant-based diet is any diet that focuses on foods derived from plant sources. This can include fruit, vegetables, grains, pulses, legumes, nuts, and meat substitutes such as soy product.[90]

A plant-based diet is based on foods derived from plants, including vegetables, whole grains, beans, nuts, seeds, and fruits, with few or no animal products.[91]

What is a Raw Plant Diet?

 Food is considered raw if it has never been heated over 104–117 °F (40–47 °C). It should also not be refined, pasteurized, treated with pesticides or otherwise processed in any way. The raw foodist uses several alternative preparation methods, such as juicing, blending processors, smart slicers, graters, slow cookers, food-dehydrating, soaking, sprouting, and low heat cooking/warming. However, some people mistakenly believe that the raw foods diet contains no cooked foods. This is not true because some raw foodists eat a diet with as little as 60% raw foods, although others will eat as much as 100%. People who are new to eating an uncooked foods diet may choose to stick to the lower end. As they realize how helpful this diet really is to their health, they may increase the amount of raw food in their diet. You will be considered a raw foodist by *Raw Food Life* if you are taking over taking over 75% uncooked food.[92]

It is also important to understand that there are different levels of being a raw plant-based foodist. Here are the choices:

- Eat a 100% raw diet that doesn't include any cooked foods at all.
- Be a raw food vegetarian in some form. Only eat plant-based foods as well as dairy and eggs.
- Eat over 75% raw plant-based and include raw milk in your diet. Use 25% cooked food in the form of cooked vegetables, starches, beans or legumes.
- Eat a partial raw foods diet. You can still be considered a raw foodist by eating as little as a 60–75% raw foods diet. This is something that

is great for a beginner, but you also may want to stick with this exclusively as you get more experienced.

To some, eating a raw food diet may sound strange. They've been accustomed to eating packaged and processed foods all their lives. It will require desire, determination, and consistency for one to change from an entirely cooked diet to having most of your food in raw form. Aside from the pure pleasure that eating raw food brings, it also gives you multiple health benefits. That is the number one reason why people end up making the switch—for their health.

The raw-food movement claims cooked food is poisonous and responsible for our ill-health and shortened lives. A recent article also stated:

> Before discovering fire, 10,000 to 20,000 years ago, we thrived for millions of years on fresh, raw, live foods furnished by nature in their whole unadulterated state. In some ways, cooking allowed humans to expand all over the world, from Africa to Antarctica. However, we paid dearly for that with shorter lifespans and many diseases.[93]

Those who follow the raw food diet believe that cooking food destroys the nutrients and the enzymes that aid digestion. What I refer here is fresh fruit, vegetables, nuts, and seeds. These are all plant-derived—not animal products. There are many potential dangers of eating raw meat. Also, care needs to be taken in the selection of raw plant-based food, to ensure wherever possible that they are organically grown and washed adequately with clean water to remove any remaining chemical residues. Raw food, especially salad, can be contaminated during preparation and hence one needs to take control.

We have a lot of foods that can be eaten in their raw form and each person needs to experiment and see what they can eat without cooking. All fruits and vegetables such as spinach, kale, lettuce, courgettes, carrots, tomatoes, chard, sprouts, celery, avocados, cabbage, etc., can be eaten without cooking. Juicing vegetables and fruits also helps to ensure you are getting more of this food in their raw form. If you feed your body with enough fruits and vegetables (raw and mildly cooked) then the other part which should consist of starches such as potatoes, rice, bread or corn can be cooked as one progress in their health journey.

Since I started writing this book, I have been surprised by all that is happening all over the world. More people are being awakened to plant food-based diets, and several doctors are now leading the change such as Dr. John Macdoughal, Dr. Fred Bisci, Dr. L. Day, Dr. T. Colin Campbell, Dr. Ellsworth Wareham, Dr. Esselstyn, and many others. Plant-based diets have always been there, but until recently many people didn't give this diet much attention. However, after realizing that we have not been able to stop many diseases—and in fact, they are on the increase, despite the rise of modern technology and research in the medical world—people are now asking questions about the food they take.

How to Transition to Raw Based Diet

When we decide to improve our diets and health, what we are really doing is learning new behaviors and turning them into habits. We are trying to break old unhealthy habits and develop new healthy ones, such as being more active and making better dietary choices. And, while there are several keys to developing a new habit, three of the most important ones are simplicity, consistency, and repetition.[94]

It is farcical, not to say pitiful, to pray to the Creator for a miraculous healing while rejecting and disregarding real divine foods, the 'fruits' of the paradise—the bread of heaven—and instead stuff your stomach three times daily with harmful prepared foods manufactured by man for commercial purposes and never destined by the Creator to be man's food at all.[95]

In order to follow a raw food diet, care needs to be taken to ensure that at least 60% of all of the food you consume is in an uncooked state (and preferably over 75%). Please note the following:

- A raw food diet can include mildly cooked vegetables, and some starches can be cooked too, such as rice, corn, or potatoes. One must be determined to increase their percentage of raw food as they progress.
- Some animal foods are allowed, such as raw milk. Some people use eggs as well.
- Eating organic food is another way to increase the benefits of the raw food diet.
- Eating a raw food diet saves you time in the kitchen because you won't need to prepare elaborate meals.

The greatest challenge when transitioning to raw foods is the desire to eat cooked food. We are addicted to cooked foods and because of the various methods of cooking with spices, salts, and oils, the foods taste delicious, and hence it is not easy to move away from this. I was able to become a vegetarian overnight but to get away from cooked food has been a difficult journey. I started by having some fruit and salad. Fruit and vegetables play a significant role in preventing vitamin C and A deficiencies. Fruits supply our bodies with potassium among other minerals. The potassium in fruit can reduce our risk of heart disease and stroke and also the risk of developing kidney stones. Potassium can also help to decrease bone loss as we age.[96]

To start a raw food diet, one does not need to make the change all at once. Changing to a raw foods diet is a personal journey.

The first step in making the switch to a raw food diet is to make sure you understand your motives for switching. At this point, it is a good idea to start a journal and talk about how you feel and why you want to make the change. Maybe you have a health problem you are hoping to solve. Or perhaps you are just doing it to be as healthy as you can.

By clearly writing down your motives, it will help keep you motivated. In a way, these motives will also become your goals. If your purpose is weight loss, for example, you can turn that into a goal by saying how many pounds you want to lose and how long you want it to take. This stage will help you begin the journey in a positive way.

As we've covered in previous chapters, raw food is just food that has not been cooked. This, however, does not mean that it needs to be completely cold. The food can actually be warmed, but just a little bit. In order for something to be classified as still raw and uncooked, it cannot be heated to anything above 117 degrees Fahrenheit. This helps in the preservation of enzymes and vitamins.

Transitioning fully to live food can be a challenge, especially when going to social places or if you have to prepare cooked food for other people. It is helpful to always carry something with you which you can eat in case of need.

Combining raw and slightly cooked food is very helpful when one is getting started. From the recommendation given by Prof. Arnold Ehret suggested in *The Mucusless Diet Healing System,* combining raw and cooked food is suitable especially for the elimination process. The ultimate aim is to able to live on more live foods as much as possible and add little cooked food to increase the bulk and fiber.

In his book, *Starch Solution,* John McDougal has emphasized the importance of complex starch in our diet.[97] I was very hesitant in the beginning because I had always associated eating carbohydrates with weight gain. When I started adding more starches into my diet, I noted an increase in energy and I didn't see any sudden increase in weight as I feared. It is true if eaten in excess that even good food can cause an increase in weight, especially if one is eating more than they are using.

Starches on their own, without adding oil, are not fattening if eaten in moderation, they make the food enjoyable and allow one to stay full without hunger issues for a longer time. The following are good starch sources: Essene bread, brown rice, sweet potatoes, oats, and oatmeal, etc. One can also make use of starchy vegetables such as green peas, beets, parsnips, winter squash, courgettes, the majority of which can be eaten raw or with mild cooking.

The following gadgets are convenient in a raw eating regime: a juicer, blender, nutribullet, food processor, hydrators, graters, smart slicers, and a slow cooker, etc.

Critics of the Raw Food Diet

Some researchers indicate that some foods are more beneficial when cooked, as they are said to release more antioxidants and are more easily digestible by the body. Some studies have shown that cooking vegetables can increase the availability of antioxidants like beta-carotene and lutein while others have found that cooking increases the antioxidant capacity and content of plant compounds found in carrots, broccoli, and zucchini. Antioxidants are important because they protect the body from harmful molecules called free radicals. The other point that is generally raised on the advantages of cooking food is that cooking food effectively kills bacteria that cause illness. However, the majority of vegetables are also very nutritious while eaten in their raw form and therefore the above statements can be very confusing for people. A combination of raw fruit and vegetables and lightly steamed vegetables can help us achieve this according to Professor Arnold in his book, *The Mucusless Diet Healing System.*[98]

I'm aware that proponents of traditional diets claim that you don't need to eat food raw in order to get nutrients since some foods get healthier when cooked. They say foods such as carrots and tomatoes release nutrients while being cooked. The other problem they cite is the possibility of exposure to bacteria and viruses in contaminated food. They say cooking and processing food get rid of harmful bacteria such as salmonella. Food poisoning can be attributed to unheated or cooked animal products, but also from fruit and vegetables that are eaten without washing.

Sometimes it can be very confusing to know who to believe. However, to get the best of two ideas, it would be therefore ideal to use raw food, carefully selected and washed and combine this with slightly cooked vegetables. Balance is the key, wherein you can integrate raw foods into your usual diet plan; but in my opinion, the majority should be in the raw form, not for a short period but as a lifestyle choice.

Why Raw Plant-Based Nutrition is Beneficial

> You must pay a high price every time you insult your body with dead and devitalized foods. Of course, you could take drugs to deaden or stimulate your body, but you are living in a fool's paradise if you think you can eat any old thing and then swallow some kind of magic pill and get away with it. You pay a dear price every time you make a garbage can of your stomach! Your heart and arteries suffer.[99]

> We just have to stop killing our food and ourselves—then we'll rediscover ourselves. Death, in the form of dead food or any other form, creates death. Life, in the form of live food or any other form, creates life. It's not profound; it's just common sense ... for a whole being! *Dead food kills. Live, raw food gives life. And the good news is you still have the Freedom to Choose.*[100]

Interestingly, I found the above statements resembling in meaning the account in the *Essene Gospel of Peace Book 1* on living foods:

> But I say to you kill neither men, nor beasts, nor yet the food which goes into your mouth. For if you eat living food, the same will quicken you, but if you kill your food, the dead food will kill you also. For life comes only from life and from death comes always death. (*Essene Gospel of Peace Book 1*)[101]

We pay dearly for our mistakes, and the scars of wrong choices remain. Can diet change help at this time? Many people chose a pill instead of a diet change because the medicine works faster. Though we still need to take medication when advised to do so by our doctors, we know there are side effects that come along with the drugs. Though we all need to see our doctors when unwell, medication is normally for a short-term, although sometimes this also can be long-term depending on the treatment. In all cases, improving our diet will help our body to respond better. Foods do not heal, but they do give our bodies and immune systems the required nutrients, vitality, and energy to enable them to do the work of healing.

Chapter 12: Enzymes

When food is cooked, most of the nutrients in the food are denatured, devitalized or destroyed altogether. Though some research says that cooking food releases nutrients, one obvious thing that happens when we cook food is that enzymes are destroyed. Cooking food with high temperatures (over 47°C/117°F) tends to destabilize some valuable enzymes and destroys certain antioxidants and vitamins. Though the body has its own in-house store of enzymes, they can be depleted with time.

> If you eat something in its natural raw state, as opposed to processing it and cooking it, I think it stands to reason that you'll get more nutrients. Your enzymes are intact. That's why I eat the way I do.[102]

One of the things that make raw foods so beneficial is that they contain enzymes. All living foods contain enzymes. In fact, our own bodies manufacture enzymes that aid digestion. For example, the enzyme lipase helps the body digest fats, and the enzyme lactase helps our bodies digest milk. Those who are lactose intolerant do not have the ability in their body to produce the lactase enzyme, mainly for genetic reasons.

No matter what our bodies need to digest, an enzyme that is produced in our bodies is a crucial part of that process. The body is equipped with different organs that help manufacture these enzymes. And even though these enzymes work throughout our lives, they slow down as we get older. This means that our bodies may not be producing all of the enzymes we need.

Since raw foods already have enzymes in them, they help relieve the pressure on our digestive systems. This, in turn, helps the digestive system work at an optimum level. It also helps the body conserve enzymes and prevents some of the drastic slow-down that the digestive system experiences as we age. However, when foods are cooked, the enzymes are largely destroyed. So, unless the food is raw, we won't get the benefit of the enzymes. Yes, we could supplement enzymes, but it is generally not a good idea to get a lot of our nutrients from supplements. Getting them from food is better for our health. The organs that make enzymes slow down as we age which means that not a lot of enzymes will always be present. If we eat raw foods, we will be better off.

Some people believe that aging is nothing more than our enzymes running out. That is another reason why people love raw food diets. It helps them maintain their youthful appearance for a lot longer. Even diets in the world that aren't necessarily raw foods focus on a lot of fresh fruits and vegetables for this reason.

Enzymes are heat sensitive and easily get deactivated when exposed to high temperatures. Nearly all enzymes are deactivated at temperatures over 47°C/117°F. *"Eat nothing therefore which a stronger fire than the fire of life has killed" (Essene Gospel of Peace Book 1).*[103] I believe fire of life refers to the natural fires such the one that ripens the fruits, and the fire within human bodies. Foods that are naturally made ready by the sun are safe as far as the enzymes are concerned, and that is why there is an emphasis on eating raw foods or those ones cooked within the above temperatures. Food hydrators and similar gadgets are useful when one is trying to add more raw foods into their regime.

According to one doctor who was a pioneer in the field of enzymes, Dr. Edward Howell, enzymes are the substances which make life possible. They are needed for every chemical reaction that occurs in our bodies. Without enzymes, no activity at all would take place, neither vitamins nor minerals nor hormones can do any work. Enzymes are complex protein molecules found in every cell in our body. They are biological catalysts which accelerate the chemical reactions in our bodies. Our bodies and all other living organisms produce their own enzymes. Enzymes are said to boost digestive work and also fight chronic diseases. A Russian study by Kazan Federal University and Voronezh University showed that some enzymes could help antibiotics and make them more effective against infections. When we eat cooked food, which is reduced in enzyme content, the body utilizes the enzymes already in our bodies to provide the needed chemical reaction. However, according to Dr. Howell, this storage is limited, and since the body's ability to manufacture enzymes diminishes as we age, our enzyme levels become depleted by over-consumption of cooked foods, stress, and illness. To compensate for the lack of food enzymes from the food we take, the body bears the full burden of producing all the enzymes for digestion of the food.[104]

Types of Enzymes and Their Sources

1. **Digestive enzymes** are created directly by the digestive system, and these are the in-house enzymes that are generated from the body's

organs. They are found in various locations throughout the gastrointestinal tract, including in the saliva, the stomach acid, the pancreatic juice, and the body's intestinal secretions.

2. **Metabolic enzymes** are produced internally and are responsible for running the body at the level of the blood, tissues, and organs. They are required for the growth of new cells and the repair and maintenance of all the body's organs and tissues.

3. **Food enzymes** are naturally present in the food we eat. Raw food contributes enzymes to the digestive process, but each brings enough to digest itself. The increased use of food enzymes promotes a decreased rate of exhaustion of the enzyme potential. Food enzymes must also have the presence of vitamins and minerals, called co-enzymes, for proper functioning. Unlike raw enzymes, co-enzymes are not entirely destroyed by cooking but are not adequately utilized when the food enzymes are destroyed.

4. **Enzyme supplementation**. Due to the inability of human beings to stick to uncooked food, there arose a need to have enzyme supplementation, and while these seem to have helped humanity, we must appreciate the best option remains raw organically grown fresh food.[105]

Aging and enzyme depletion go hand in hand, and by restoring vital enzymes, Howell proposes we can live longer and healthier lives.

> The increased use of food enzymes promotes a decreased rate of exhaustion of the enzyme potential. Any kind of raw diet cuts down enzyme secretion and gives the enzyme machinery a rest…. Enzymes offer an important means of calculating the vital energy of an organism. That which has been referred to as vitality, vital force, vital energy, vital activity, nerve energy, nerve force, strength, vital resistance, life energy, life, and life force, maybe, and probably is, synonymous with that which has been known as enzyme activity, enzyme value, enzyme energy, enzyme vitality, and enzyme content. For every aspect of life and personality are enzyme-driven, enzyme dependent. Life is an enzyme process.[106]

This agrees with the ideas contained in the *Essene Gospel of Peace Book 1*:

> For the power of God's angels enters into you with the living food which the Lord gives you from his royal table.[107]

We've discussed that raw foods have a lot of health benefits. These health benefits are what bring people to the diet in the first place. The following are some of these health benefits.

Raw foods help to increase energy. One thing that the raw foods diet is known for is to help people feel more energetic. When the body is being fed the right balance of nutrients and enzymes, it makes our body systems function even better. The reward is that everything will run more efficiently which will then improve our energy levels.

The modern diet, especially one that is filled with processed foods, depletes our energy levels because of the toll it takes on our digestive system. The raw foods diet helps this because it adds the enzymes and other nutrients back into your body.

You see, our bodies are meant to function a certain way when fed all the right nutrients. This is what makes the raw foods diet so powerful. The body has a chance to work at its optimal level because, with a raw foods diet, you are giving it the nutrients that it needs.

> Raw food may help improve health against heart disease. Heart disease is a big problem in our modern society. Poor diet and lack of exercise add to the problem and even cause the problem in most people. If we were to take the time to care for our bodies by exercising and eating right, then heart disease risk would be greatly reduced.[108]

The raw foods diet helps you look your best because it contains a good balance of nutrients to help keep your skin, hair, and nails looking fresh and healthy. The skin is especially affected because if the body is filled with toxins and unhealthy byproducts, it will show on the skin. Since a raw foods diet is detoxifying and not harmful, the skin will clear up. Also, hair will become shinier, and the nails will grow stronger.

Weight loss is a big thing when it comes to the raw plant-based diet because the food is low in fat and calories. This means that one will lose weight while following the diet. Weight loss is one of the most desirable benefits of these diets especially because it comes naturally.

People who follow the raw foods diet will also experience improved digestion. This has a lot to do with the enzymes, but it is also because of the relatively high fiber content of the diet. The modern Western diet depletes the digestive system and causes it to work too hard. Since the raw foods diet contains enzymes of its own, the digestive system doesn't need to release a lot of its own enzymes. This leads to greater efficiency within the digestive system. If the digestive system isn't working correctly, it can really take a toll on your health.

Overall, the raw food diet improves your overall state of health, mainly because of the high nutrient content of the diet but also because of the enzymes. Once the body has the nutrients it needs, all of the body systems will begin to function a lot better. The increased energy that happens because of this growing efficiency helps to improve the body's general health, especially over a more extended time period such as several months or even several years.

Chapter 13: Noted Health Conditions

The purpose of this section is to highlight some of the conditions that led me to search for answers and hence led me to a lifestyle change. However, what is written is for information only and is not medical advice. Please consult your doctor for any medical advice.

The conditions I would like to explore in this chapter include cardiovascular diseases, some types of autoimmune disorders such as Alopecia Universalis, thyroid issues, acid reflux, diabetes, eczema, and arthritis.

People suffer from various conditions in their lives, and though I may not be able to mention everyone's condition, one thing that is common with all sicknesses is its source. The source is either, as said before, due to toxin overload, nutrition deficiency, acids, inflammation, blockage of the lymphatic system, and generally body system breakdown. All diseases come from the same source only being manifested in areas of weakness.

Cardiovascular Diseases

I still remember those dreadful phone calls informing me of the sudden demise of close members of my family. When as a family we learned about the death of my brother, we were devastated to the core. As a firstborn, my brother acted as a father to his young siblings since our dad lived far away from us. It was also common for the firstborn, whether boys or girls, to play the role of a parent to the other siblings. That was the case with my brother and later my sister.

It has been over 25 years since this happened, but I'm still searching for answers. Probably this would not have been the case had it not been followed by the same fate befalling my sister and later another brother. The death of my siblings (the last one being in 2015) accelerated my search for health which I had already started, but I was not sure what I needed to know. What we were told is that the three siblings died of cardiovascular diseases that caused heart attacks. This is one of the reasons that I would like to write on this disease—to give some insight to people who are looking for answers. As mentioned, this is for information only and the best person suited to provide personal medical advice is your doctor.

The first time I heard of cardiovascular disease I was in high school when one of my classmates received the news that her dad had died of a heart attack.

We were too young to accurately understand what that meant, but we understood that he had died suddenly. It was many years ago, but I still remember the pain on the girl's face as she realized her dad would no longer be able to drop her off in school. Years later, when my own siblings died of the same problem, I still didn't know much about the connection between diet and heart disease, but I started to ask questions. I can't claim to say I know much now, but I wish to create an awareness for people that nutrition is the key to managing heart disease. From my research, I believe that a change of lifestyle that includes diet, exercise, weight management, and supplementation, is the key to overcoming this disease, in conjunction (not instead of) other treatments and monitoring by the doctor.

The main drawback of cardiovascular disease is that the majority of people do not know they have a problem until something goes wrong and by then for many people, it is too late. Most people have little or no warning, and if no medical intervention is made within the shortest period, the experience can be devastating. The majority of people do not know how to give CPR (cardiopulmonary resuscitation) and hence cannot help anyone suffering a heart attack. Other people live also where no ambulance services are available, and there are no plans in place for when such a thing happens (I'm referring here to some places in developing countries like Kenya where I grew up). Therefore, it's important for everyone to know how to take care of themselves, by avoiding the disease altogether or doing what is in your power to do.

However, the thought that a man's life can disappear suddenly without notice is quite frightening. It gives a sense of desperation like humanity is doomed, having to work so hard, struggle in life, and then suddenly disappear.

In my helplessness, I related to the Essene people's cry for help from the master, Jesus. "Oh Lord help your people they need an answer, we don't know what to do," I cried. During my brother's autopsy, my mother was in the room, and she explained to me that she saw indications of an unhealthy lifestyle. As we are going to see later, there are some factors that they call modifiable and unmodifiable factors that may be to blame for this devastating disease.

Diet and lifestyle change can go a long way in helping people have a healthier body and healthier cardiovascular system.

The scriptures tell us that due to lack of knowledge people perish (see Hosea 4:6a). Equally, we may have the knowledge and yet refuse to obey or listen because we are too busy with life, too busy making ends meet to sit down and ask ourselves some serious health questions.

> But if they do not listen, they perish by the sword and die without knowledge. (*Job 36:12*)

All over the world, a vast number of people have left this Earth prematurely due to cardiovascular diseases. Though eventually everyone, even if we reach 120 years, will leave this world, cardiovascular deaths are sudden and often present little warning. Families and loved ones are left devastated, dreams and plans are shattered, so many tasks left unaccomplished. Cardiovascular diseases are not easy to determine, and problems can build over time without our being aware of them.

Cardiovascular disease is the silent killer because if no help is received immediately when a problem shows up, death can quickly occur.

What is Cardiovascular Disease?

Every part of the body needs oxygen and nutrients to stay alive, and it's our cardiovascular system that accomplishes this task for all the years that we are breathing and alive. Our cardiovascular system, as we all know from our biology, is made up of the heart and the blood vessels. The blood vessels consist of arteries, veins, and capillaries. The arteries take oxygenated blood with the help of capillaries further as it flows to the entire body. The veins carry oxygen-depleted blood back to the heart for replenishing, and the whole process continues until our last breath. Most of us did some science at school, and we could describe the functioning of the heart and how the blood flows to and from the heart to the body. Yet I wonder how many of us carry that knowledge with us to help us live healthy lives. If you are like me, I did it to pass an exam. As we grow older and become busy with life, we become ignorant of this great engine within us that is very crucial for our survival. We become complacent in everything we eat and do. We abdicate our health responsibility to the physicians; after all, we are not doctors, and we can't understand our bodies, we say. In fact, some people don't dare read medical journals because they think they can't understand them. And yet this great system is still within us. We need to have some understanding of how it works and how we can support it to work more efficiently and with less disturbance.

Most people are not engineers or mechanics, but they know how to maintain their cars and other gadgets. How surprising, then, that they have so little interest in the engine inside them. I know I have been one such person, very much unaware of the effects of my food and lifestyle on this vital organ.

Unfortunately, our diligent workaholic cardiovascular system does not complain even when things are not too good and always looks for ways to work even under adverse conditions, sometimes sending signs and signals to say all is not well, but we fail to recognize them in good time or just ignore them as pains and probably take some pain killers.

However, with all its struggles it reaches a stage where it is unable to function, due to lack of oxygenated blood and nutrients, etc. Without warning, people experience symptoms that require sudden attention. Otherwise, they may suffer heart attacks or strokes and if there is no immediate external help death may take place.

The primary cardiovascular diseases are atherosclerosis (coronary heart disease), coronary artery disease, high blood pressure, and stroke.

Atherosclerosis (Coronary Heart Disease)

When people are young their arteries are cleaner and flexible, but as they age, this flexibility is reduced, and the artery accumulates fatty deposits or arterial plaque, a condition known as atherosclerosis.

According to the British Heart Foundation, coronary heart disease (CHD) is the most common form of cardiovascular disease. It is when the arteries supplying the heart with oxygen-rich blood become narrowed by the gradual build-up of fatty materials in their walls. The fatty substance is called atheroma or arterial plaque, and this causes, among other things, damage to the endothelium (the cells which line the interior surface of blood vessels and lymphatic vessels).

As we already know, arteries are blood vessels which carry oxygenated blood throughout the body. This activity can be affected if they are clogged due to the build-up of plaque on the inside walls. The build-up of plaque can reduce blood flow or block it altogether, and when this happens, the likelihood of getting a heart attack or stroke is high. In the same way, if a piece of atheroma/plaque breaks off and gets dislodged from the walls of the artery, the body responds by causing the blood to clot, and if this remains untreated it will prevent the oxygen-rich blood from reaching the heart or the brain, and this may also cause a heart attack or stroke.

Clogged arteries or plaque in the arteries in various parts of the body may lead to conditions such as mentioned below.

- **Coronary artery disease.** This affects the arteries carrying oxygenated rich blood to the heart. This condition frequently gives no warning until symptoms appear suddenly and require immediate medical attention. Symptoms may show up as chest pains and shortness of breath, among others. The oxygenated blood is blocked from entering the heart due to the build-up of plaque or due to a blood clot. Either of these will lower or completely prevent the oxygenated blood full of nutrients from entering the heart; when this happens, a partial or a complete heart attack may take place.
- **Carotid artery diseases.** Carotid arteries run on either side of the neck, and they supply oxygen to the brain. When plaque accumulates in these arteries, or a clot is formed, the rich oxygenated blood is wholly or partially blocked from reaching the brain. When such a thing happens, a partial or complete stroke takes place. Sometimes it can be mild, but it can sometimes lead to paralysis (temporary or permanent) or even death. Both heart attack and stroke have the same causes, only that one attacks happens in the heart and the other in the brain.
- **Periphery artery diseases.** This is the disease of the vessels that carry blood to the legs. The build-up of plaque in this region may cause numbness, pains, and infections in the legs and feet.

Heart Attack

As discussed in the previous section, when a piece of atheroma/plaque breaks off and get dislodged from the walls of the artery, the body responds by causing the blood to clot. If this is not treated or dissolved in time, it will prevent the oxygen-rich blood from reaching the heart and may cause a heart attack which can be irreversible or fatal. Heart attacks may also be caused by the build-up of plaque which restricts the flow of blood to the heart. It is said that sudden contraction can also occur in the arteries which would equally deprive the heart of oxygen suddenly with the same devastating effects. Some of the symptoms are intense pain in the chest, pain radiating down the arms, shoulder or neck, shortness of breath, nausea, light-headedness, dizziness, anxiety, and fatigue among others. With early and quick intervention many people survive heart attacks.

Lowering the blood pressure and cholesterol, healthy diet, and exercise are some of the things that people can do to help themselves reduce the risk. Regular medical check-ups are crucial in managing medication conditions such as blood pressure, cholesterol levels, and other important health indicators.

Hypertension/High Blood Pressure

Hypertension is a long-term medical condition in which the blood pressure in the arteries is persistently elevated. Hypertension, also known as raised blood pressure, is a significant risk factor for cardiovascular diseases. When the volume of blood is too high for the vessels, the elevated blood pressure increases the workload on the heart, which in turn damages the blood vessels. High blood pressure, just like the other cardiovascular diseases, is also caused by the constriction of the arteries which restrict the flow of blood.

The deadly problem with high blood pressure is that because it is silent, one can't feel it. Yet despite this lack of physical symptoms, it may inwardly be causing damage to the endothelium, which may eventually lead to atherosclerosis and atheroma formation and the outcome may be the same as that of other cardiovascular diseases. High blood pressure is a significant risk factor for coronary artery disease, stroke, heart failure, peripheral vascular disease, vision loss, and chronic kidney disease. People with high blood pressure also report headaches, particularly at the back of the head.

Risk Factors for Hypertension

The risk of developing high blood pressure increases as you get older, or if you have a family history of high blood pressure, being of African or Caribbean origin, a high amount of salt in your food, a lack of exercise, being overweight or obese, regularly drinking large amounts of alcohol, smoking, or long-term sleep deprivation. Maintaining correct levels of cholesterol is vital for the maintenance of healthy arteries. We know this is a challenge to so many people. Of greater importance is to ensure your LDL is not elevated and your total cholesterol is within limits. Having a diet with low saturated fats and trans fats etc., and being physically active, while consuming foods that will provide good fats to the body such as Omega 3, are some of the ways to ensure that the levels are kept within limits.

Stroke

The blockage of the arteries can trigger stroke, but this time the arteries involved are those that run at both side of the neck. When the blood clots in the vessels leading to the brain, they prevent the normal flow of blood, and they deprive the brain cells of oxygen and nutrients leading to a stroke which can lead to brain damage, physical disability, and sometimes death. The risk factors are the same as for other cardiovascular diseases.

Leading Causes of Atherosclerosis/Coronary Heart Diseases/Coronary Artery Disease

We understand there are two main risks or causes of the above disease: unmodifiable risks factors and modifiable risks factors.

Unmodifiable Risks

These are risks mainly related to age, gender, and family history.

Age. As people age the risks of having a cardiovascular disease increase. This is because the arteries stop being as flexible as they were before and with age the arteries are bound to have slowly accumulated more plaque from the blood, hence causing a build-up.

Gender. They say men more than women suffer more from cardiovascular disease due to a lack of protective estrogen, though many women suffer from the condition.

Family history. This could be due to an individual's genotype (the genetic constitution of an individual organism).

One of the possibilities of why there is a history of these diseases in a family could be due to lipid metabolism.

Lipidosis

Fats (lipids) are an essential source of energy for the body. The body's store of fat is continuously broken down and reassembled to balance the body's energy needs with the food available. Groups of specific enzymes help the body break down and process fats. Specific abnormalities in these enzymes can lead to the build-up of specific fatty substances that typically would have been broken down by the enzymes. Over time, accumulations of these substances can be harmful to many organs of the body. Disorders caused by the accumulation of lipids are called lipidoses. Other enzyme abnormalities prevent the body from converting fats into energy normally. These abnormalities are called fatty acid oxidation disorders.[109]

A lipid storage disorder (or lipidosis) can be any one of a group of inherited metabolic disorders in which harmful amounts of fats or lipids accumulate in some of the body's cells and tissues. People with these disorders either do not produce enough of one of the enzymes needed to metabolize and break down lipids or they produce enzymes that do not work properly.[110]

Our body uses fat (lipids) as a vital source of energy. This form of fat is derived from the food we eat. A group of specific enzymes helps the body break down the fat into energy but due to specific abnormalities in these enzymes this process is not done efficiently, and there arises a build-up of fatty substances in the organs of the body leading to lipidosis which is a disorder of lipid accumulation.

Fatty Acid Oxidation Disorder

An abnormality called fatty acid oxidation disorder occurs due to other enzyme abnormalities which also prevent the body from converting fats into energy as is supposed to be the case.

Fatty acid oxidation is a broad classification for genetic disorders that result from an inability of the body to produce or utilize one enzyme that is required to oxidize fatty acids. The enzyme can be missing or improperly constructed, resulting in it not working. This leaves the body unable to produce energy within the liver and muscles from fatty acid sources. The body's primary source of energy is glucose; however, when all the glucose in the body has been expended, a normal body digests fat. Individuals with a fatty-acid metabolism disorder are unable to metabolize this fat source for energy, halting bodily processes. Most individuals with a fatty-acid metabolism disorder can live a healthy active life with simple adjustments to diet and medication.[111]

There is nothing much you can do about your family history, and if you have a family history of cardiovascular disease may mean you are exposed to the kind of risk factor that you can't change.[112]

> Your genes and your family disease history are like a loaded gun. Your lifestyle choices dictate whether you pull the trigger or not. (Annette Larkins)[113]

It is true that though you can't change your family's background, you can drastically reduce your risk of getting cardiovascular disease by changing your lifestyle and controlling other risk factors.

> Our data indicates even those with strong family history when eating plant-based diets are protected from vascular disease. Family history loads the gun, but lifestyle pulls the trigger. (Dr. Esselstyn)[114]

Uses of Vegetables and Fruit

There is compelling evidence that a diet rich in fruits and vegetables can lower the risk of heart disease and stroke. The largest and longest study was done as part of the Harvard-based Nurses' Health Study and Health Professionals Follow-up Study, included almost 10,000 men and women whose health and dietary habits were followed for 14 years and the results confirmed the benefits of a diet of fruits and vegetables towards cardiovascular health.

When researchers combined findings from the Harvard studies with several other long-term studies in the US and Europe and looked at coronary heart disease and stroke separately, they found a similar protective effect. Individuals who ate more than 5 servings of fruits and vegetables per day had roughly a 20% lower risk of coronary heart disease and stroke (compared with individuals who consumed less than 3 servings per day).

> We should all be eating fruits and vegetables as if our lives depend on it – because they do. (Michael Greger)[115]

To promote our cardiovascular health, we need to incorporate a diet of fruits and vegetables. To get the maximum benefits, these should be used in their raw form. Since it's not easy to take enough vegetables in the raw form, especially the leafy ones, adding vegetable juice to your regime will help ensure you are taking enough vegetables. Some of the vegetables can be lightly steamed, but the greater portion of the vegetables need to be in the raw form. Fruits are the easiest to take, though many people worry about the fruit's sugar. We need to by-pass the sugar fears and see the overall benefits that eating fruit provides, besides the sugar content.

Fruit is loaded with vitamins, minerals, antioxidants, and fiber so it can be incredibly beneficial for our bodies; but try to limit those higher in sugars, choose fresh over dried and eat whole fruits rather than just drinking their juice. Nutritionist Fiona Hunter says: "The idea that fruit is the enemy is fuelled by the current preoccupation with sugar but looking at one nutrient in isolation, without considering what else a food brings, is a real mistake."[116] Fruit (and veg) provide a host of phytochemicals and there is a growing body of evidence to suggest that these phytochemicals can protect against a whole host of health problems including certain types of cancer, heart disease, cataracts, and dementia so cutting fruit out of your diet because you are worried about sugar is like throwing out the baby with the bath water.[117]

Instead of avoiding fruit because of sugar, it is better to cut off other sugar sources especially the added sugars and white flour.

Managing your weight. Trying to get into your normal or natural weight is helpful because it reduces weight burden from the body and in most cases, it means you will experience fat loss although in some cases this is not the case.

Not smoking or stopping smoking. As explained smoking is a risk factor to all the cardiovascular diseases and hence when one quits smoking it means there is a great improvement towards one's health.

Ensuring your blood pressure is normal. High blood pressure is a risk factor for many diseases not only cardiovascular disease and hence keeping it low is a step towards health improvement.

Saturated fats. Saturated fat is blamed for causing high LDL cholesterol which is one of the causes of atherosclerosis. The primary source of saturated fats is animal products. It's well known that animal products, such as dairy products, beef, mutton, and poultry have saturated fat and hence are contributory factors to bad cholesterol.

The relationship between cardiovascular risk and blood cholesterol levels have been demonstrated from large studies. Low-density lipoprotein (LDL) cholesterol is classed as a dominant risk factor for cardiovascular disease while HDL (high-density lipoprotein) helps in lowering the bad cholesterol. Therefore, our concern should be to try to reduce our bad cholesterol while increasing our good cholesterol. Once you get your levels checked you will be able to know what action you need to take.

In his study *China Study*, T. Colin Campbell found out that it's not only the saturated fat in cow's milk that is bad for our health but also the milk casein.[118] However, as I said before, it's not clear from his studies whether he differentiated between casein from raw and unpasteurized milk and between A1 and A2 casein. However, I have not done extensive research like T. Campbell so it's good to follow the word of the experts in case you have a chronic illness that you suspect milk casein could be a culprit.

Use of Oils

Another new positive piece of information that I learned during my research while writing this book was about oils. My concern previously was to minimize saturated fats and increase use of good fats in moderation. However, after reading the work of Dr. Esselstyn, I was astonished to learn that even the oils I thought were beneficial are really not that good.[119] **No oils!** Not even olive oil, which goes against a lot of other advice out there about so-called good fats. The reality is that oils are extremely low in terms of nutritional value. They contain no fiber, no minerals and are 100% fat calories. Both the monounsaturated and saturated fat contained in oils is harmful to the endothelium, the innermost lining of the artery, and that injury is the gateway to vascular disease. It doesn't matter whether it's olive oil, corn oil, coconut oil, canola oil, or any other kind. Avoid ALL oil.[120]

The non-use of oils, especially vegetable oils, has been echoed by other doctors such as Dr. John McDougal in his book *Starch Solution*.[121]

The above information amazed me. I believed in olive oil, and I have been trying to get the purest of them all, raw cold pressed virgin oil. I was shocked to note that I don't need to add any extracted oil to my foods. The oils are to be consumed in their original form, but once extracted their food value changes. The food we eat, vegetables, grains, and fruits all have their own oils to help them be digested. One will, however, need to eat a balanced diet, to ensure they are getting oil naturally especially the Omega 3 fatty acids from food. Foods such as flaxseeds (flax needs to be ground) or chia seeds are well tolerated and supply a bonus of Omega 3. Nuts such as almonds, walnuts, Brazil nuts can be used sparingly but are best in their raw form. Spirulina and chlorella are also good sources of Omega 3 for vegans and vegetarians.

There are contradicting reports on the usage of oils such as olive and coconut oils, and one may require doing further research to determine what is right for them.

In conclusion, we know fat plays a significant role in the body. Therefore we need to include a small amount of it in our diet. The best source is getting the fat or oil straight from its source instead of using the extracted form, e.g., from an avocado, nut, seeds, seaweeds such as spirulina, chlorella for the vegetarians and vegans. Fat fulfills a wide range of functions, in our body which include:

- Supplying energy for cells.
- Fat provides essential fatty acids which the body is not able to make.
- Some vitamins, A, D, E, and K are fat-soluble, and fats help in their transportation.
- Fat is useful in hormone production and provides a protective layer around vital organs.

Fat is very high in calories with each gram of fat providing more than twice as many calories compared to protein and carbohydrate. One gram of fat contains nine calories while protein and carbohydrates provide four calories each.

When it comes to fat, the type also matters. Having too much saturated fat in our diet can cause high levels of bad cholesterol LDL which can increase the risk of cardiovascular disease.

Nitric Oxide

In my reading and research on the cardiovascular diseases I came across the book by Dr. Louis J. Ignarro, *No More Heart Diseases*.

From his work, I learned in depth about nitric oxide and the role it plays in ensuring cardiovascular health and the things we need to do to boost its production in our bodies.

Nitric oxide is a molecular chemical compound which has received a good deal of attention due to its cardiovascular benefits. It is an important regulator and mediator of numerous processes in the nervous, immune, and cardiovascular systems. These include vascular smooth muscle relaxation, resulting in arterial vasodilation (the dilatation of blood vessels, which decreases blood pressure), and increasing blood flow.

As a consequence of its importance in neuroscience, physiology, and immunology, nitric oxide was proclaimed "Molecule of the Year" in 1992. Research into its function led to the 1998 Nobel Prize for discovering the role of nitric oxide as a cardiovascular signaling molecule[122] being given to Robert F. Furchgott, Ferid Murad and Louis J. Ignarro.

The interior surface of the arteries (endothelium) produces nitric oxide, and when plaque builds up in the arteries, a condition known as atherosclerosis, it reduces the capacity of the endothelium to produce nitric oxide. Emerging evidence seems to suggest that coronary artery disease is related to defects in the generation of nitric oxide.

Boosting nitric oxide is extraordinarily good at preventing cardiovascular disease, as it relaxes arterial walls, dilates the vessels, and improves the flow of blood.[123]

Therefore, increasing nitric oxide makes the body run more efficiently, as oxygen, nutrients, and red blood cells can reach their target tissue and cells more quickly.

How to Increase Nitric Oxide in Our Body

According to many studies and particularly the one conducted by Dr. Louis J. Ignarro, a Nobel Laureate in Medicine, the following amino acids and vitamins supplements among others seem to enhance the production of nitric oxide in the human body. These are L-arginine, L-citrulline, vitamin C, vitamin E, folic acid and alpha lipoic acid. For the dosage amount, please seek help from your health adviser. In his book, Dr. Louis J. Ignarro has given details on how to use these supplements.

Other studies have shown the importance of sunshine in the production of nitric oxide, though it's not very clear whether supplementation with vitamin D3 would help in winter seasons. Several studies have also found out that pycnogenol increases nitric oxide, improves blood flow, and reduces the symptoms of venous leakage.[124]

Point of caution, one should always check with their medical doctors to ensure they can use the supplements and especially if they are on other medication. Vitamin E which has blood-thinning properties should not be taken in conjunction with blood thinning medicines unless under a doctor's supervision or advice.

Exercise

We have already discussed exercise in a previous chapter. I believe any form of regular exercise that is suitable for an individual will help in increasing the production of nitric oxide in the body and support the whole-body function.

Nutrition

A diet of fruit, vegetables, whole grains, and seeds would also support the production of nitric oxide. Avoiding saturated fats is recommended because this increases the LDL levels that may cause a build-up of plaque in the arteries thereby reducing the levels of nitric oxide. According to Ignarro, some of the food groups that would help in nitric oxide production are fruits and vegetables, whole grains, brown rice, beans and peas, flaxseeds, fiber, nuts, and seeds. Fruits such as grapes, blueberries, and pomegranate are the best source of polyphenols and antioxidants and support nitric oxide production.

Autoimmune Diseases

Autoimmune disease disorder is a wide area, and I have no intention of covering it in detail in this book. Some conditions, such Alopecia Universalis, acid reflux, thyroid problems, leaky gut issues, diabetes, eczema and a number of other diseases are said to be as a result of immunity disorder.

According to diabetes.co.uk, autoimmune disease develops when your body's immune system treats healthy cells in your body as foreign cells and attacks them. Autoimmune diseases are disorders that occur when healthy tissue (cells) get destroyed by the body's own immune system. There are more than 80 different types of autoimmune disease, from multiple sclerosis and type 1 diabetes to coeliac disease and rheumatoid arthritis.

According to Dr. Hyman of Dr. Hyman.com, autoimmune conditions are connected by one central biochemical process; a runaway immune response also known as systemic inflammation that results in your body attacking its own tissues.

According to Diabetes UK, the exact cause of autoimmune disease is unknown, although there are many theories about what causes it to malfunction including:

- Bacteria or virus, drugs, chemical irritants, environmental irritants.
- Studies have shown that autoimmune disorders often run in families and are much more common in women.
- Leaky gut. [125]

Autoimmune Disease Treatment

While there are no cures for autoimmune disorders, there are various methods of treating them, depending on the type of disease. Ways of achieving this include the following among many others:

- Living a healthy lifestyle. That includes eating a healthy balanced diet, exercising regularly, reducing stress, and getting plenty of rest.
- Getting checked for heavy metal toxicity.
- Getting tested for celiac disease.
- By fixing the gut issues.
- Make use of nutrients such as Omega 3, vitamin C, and probiotics, etc.
- Getting checked for hidden infections, yeast, virus, bacteria, etc.
- Use of medication as recommended by the doctor—including pain relievers, anti-inflammatory drugs (if joints are affected), and immunosuppressive medication.
- Avoiding any known causes of flare-ups.

Leaky Gut

Leaky gut, or "intestinal permeability," is a condition in which the lining of the small intestine becomes damaged, causing undigested food particles, toxic waste products, and bacteria to "leak" through the intestines and flood the bloodstream. The foreign substances entering the blood can cause an autoimmune response in the body including inflammatory and allergic reactions such as migraines, irritable bowel, eczema, chronic fatigue, food allergies, rheumatoid arthritis, and more. With leaky gut, damaged cells in your intestines don't produce the enzymes needed for proper digestion. As a result, your body cannot absorb essential nutrients, which can lead to hormone imbalances and a weakened immune system. [126]

Having leaky gut is kind of like having the gates broken from your intestines to your bloodstream.[127] The following are some possible causes of a leaky gut:

Poor diet. People react differently to different foods, and we all need to take action when our bodies respond to certain foods, either avoiding them or keeping away from them for a while to see what happens. Test for allergies and check to see which food causes trouble. Fruit, vegetables, and whole carbohydrates cause little or no intestinal problems if they are organically produced. The problem with non-organic fruit and vegetables is the potential for them to have pesticides and chemical residues, one of the possible causes of leaky gut. Foods to be avoided to overcome leaky gut syndrome include all animal proteins, gluten, and unsprouted grains.

Chronic stress. It is difficult to avoid stress, but there are many ways one can try to manage stressful moments in life. Exercise (walking, gym), music, prayer, and meditation are helpful in managing stress. Also, getting involved in the community and helping where you can will engage your thoughts with other matters outside those of your own.

Toxin overload. One can take a toxicology test to help discover the cause of certain conditions. Using organically produced food, less use of antibiotics, and pain killers such as NSAIDS will start one on a journey towards healing. However, it's not easy, as it takes time to remove all the toxins from the body. Water and juice fasting will help accelerate the healing process as mentioned in the fasting chapter.

Bacterial imbalance. Making use of probiotics will help overcome the bacterial imbalance while limiting the use of antibiotics.

Some other causes mentioned elsewhere in the literature include molds, metal toxicity, and parasites.

Symptoms of Leaky Gut

According to Dr. Leo Galland, director of the Foundation for Integrated Medicine, the following symptoms might be signs of leaky gut: chronic diarrhea, constipation, gas or bloating, nutritional deficiencies, weak immune system, headaches, brain fog, memory loss, excessive fatigue, skin rashes and problems such as acne, eczema or rosacea, cravings for sugar or carbs, arthritis or joint pain, depression, anxiety, ADHD, autoimmune diseases such as rheumatoid arthritis, lupus, celiac disease or Crohn's disease.

He further says the key to healing a leaky gut is changing one's diet and eliminating the foods that your body treats as toxic, adding those that will help you recover. Supplements such as probiotics and amino acid L-glutamine are said to be helpful towards the healing process.

Others included by Dr. Axe are thyroid disease, food sensitivities, inflammatory bowel disease, nutrient malabsorption, inflammatory skin conditions, mood issues, autism, and Alopecia (Areata, Totalis and Universalis).

The following is what the NHS UK states:

> While it's true that some conditions and medications can cause a "leaky" gut (what scientists call increased intestinal permeability), there is currently little evidence to support the theory that a porous bowel is the direct cause of any significant, widespread problems. There is also little evidence that the "treatments" which some people claim help to reduce bowel leakiness, such as nutritional supplements and herbal remedies, have any beneficial effect for most of the conditions they supposedly help.[128]

How to Heal a Leaky Gut

The key to healing a leaky gut is changing one's diet and eliminating the foods that the body treats as a toxin. The best way is to try and remove all the foods you identify as causing the problem. Visiting a nutritionist who will be able to do an allergy test may be a good starting point. Check for hidden food allergens with IgG food testing, which is designed to eliminate most food allergens and avoid triggers.

Replacing the food you have a reaction to with the healing foods of organically produced raw fruit and vegetables, sprouted grains, and raw milk may help. Maintain a diet of more than 5 servings of fruit and vegetables a day.

Despite the NHS advice, there are various supplements which are suggested by some to be useful in supporting gut health. These include digestive enzymes, probiotics, L-glutamine, licorice root, quercetin (DGL), vitamins C, D, E and Omega 3 among others. Always consult your doctor or health advisers before embarking on the use of supplements.

Most health experts recommend the use of probiotics to balance out gut flora. Seek advice from your health adviser to know which one is best suited for you. Doing your own research can help you also on this journey. Get tested for celiac disease, too (this is a disease in which the small intestine is hypersensitive to gluten, leading to difficulty in digesting food).

Check for hidden infection. With the help of a doctor, check for yeast, viruses, or bacteria and get treated if an infection is found. Some people have claimed healing when hidden infections were treated.

Get checked for heavy metal toxicity. Mercury and other metals can cause autoimmunity. One can also include chlorella supplements. One claimed benefit includes its ability to protect the body against toxic metals such as lead and mercury.

Exercise regularly. Exercise is beneficial for the whole-body system, and it is a natural anti-inflammatory.

Alopecia Universalis

Alopecia Universalis is a condition characterized by the complete loss of hair on the scalp and body. It is an advanced form of Alopecia Areata, a condition that causes round patches of hair loss. Although the exact cause is unknown, it is thought to be an autoimmune disorder in which the person's immune system mistakenly attacks the hair follicles. There is currently no cure for Alopecia Universalis, though they say sometimes hair regrowth can occur on its own, even after many years.

This is one of the major problems I have endured for many years. When my hair started showing problems, I had no knowledge of the effects of food on my overall health, neither did the doctors I approached mention anything to do with nutrition. Most of my treatments were topical on the scalp or the hair. I tried various oils and shampoos, none of which helped, and I eventually lost my hair.

Though I have not experienced regrowth, I felt I needed to talk about this to help those who have started to see trouble with their hair. Prevention is better than cure, and one doesn't need to see symptoms before they embark on a healthy lifestyle. It took me many years to accept my hair loss and new look. The real cause of my hair loss is still unknown to me, but when I look back in the past, I tend to think it was a combination of various factors, such as poor nutrition, medication, trauma, stress, emotional disturbance, etc.

Most people are not aware of this severe condition. Sometimes it goes unnoticed because the victims of the disease cover up with either wigs or hats. It looks harmless, but it is not an easy condition for the victim. It takes away people's confidence, and without proper care and counseling, this can lead to other conditions such as self-pity, rejection, low esteem, and even depression.

When my hair condition started to become worse, I was referred to a specialist who diagnosed the problem as Alopecia Universalis and was started on treatment for over a year, but unfortunately, it didn't work. It was very a lonely and depressing journey. Today there are many support groups that help people with this condition, such as Alopecia UK.

What was concerning me during my struggle with hair was my outside looks and I was definitely ignorant of the internal underlying causes and the nutritional factor. After more than 10 years of suffering, that is when I started to wonder whether my diet had something to do with my hair loss and by then I had developed other conditions such as food sensitivities, acid reflux, and other similar conditions that awoke my interest in health through nutrition. For those who are in the early stages of Alopecia or simple hair loss, my advice to you is to immediately embark on a healthy diet as suggested in this book.

Current Research with Hope on Hair Loss

While there is currently no treatment capable of completely restoring hair, there are several recent studies showing that a class of medication known as JAK inhibitors, which includes Tofacitinib and Ruxolitinib, are effective in the treatment of Alopecia Areata, including Alopecia Universalis. However, JAK inhibitors have not yet been approved by the FDA for use in skin conditions.

"Although our study was small, it provides crucial evidence that JAK inhibitors may constitute the first effective treatment for people with Alopecia Areata," says Dr. Julian Mackay-Wiggan, associate professor of dermatology and director of the Clinical Research Unit in the Department of Dermatology at CUMC, and a dermatologist at New York-Presbyterian/Columbia. "This is encouraging news for patients who are coping with the physical and emotional effects of this disfiguring autoimmune disease," she adds.[129]

Previous research by the team revealed specific immune cells and dominant inflammatory signaling pathways that are responsible for attacking the hair follicles in people with Alopecia Areata, resulting in the follicle entering a dormant state. Later studies of mouse and human hair follicles showed that JAK inhibitors reawaken these dormant follicles by blocking inflammatory signaling.

By the time I'm writing this book, this treatment is not yet available in the UK, but I hope this, and others yet to be discovered, will help people who are suffering from this disfiguring autoimmune disease. It is especially terrible for women and girls whose hair is considered as beauty. I struggled with my hair for more than 12 years, and you can imagine the mental anguish, the emotional disturbance, the money, and the time consumed in trying to get the hair back. It reminded me of the story of the woman in the Bible (Luke 8:40–48) who endured the issue of blood and spent her money for 12 years. Her story ended well when she was healed, and therefore all things are possible; even the most difficult problems can be overcome—like hair loss.

How to Manage Hair Loss for Women

For women, there's a social stigma attached to going bald and losing your hair can severely affect your confidence and how you perceive yourself. Many people find it difficult to disclose their hair loss to family members and friends, and for this reason, they struggle to find answers to their condition on their own. If one has lost hair or is losing hair, it is advisable to discuss this situation with family and friends so that they can be part of your journey and can give support when you need it.

It is also essential to address the psychological impact of hair loss, and life will be easier if you can accept what's happened and learn to live with your altered appearance, but this depends on one's coping strategy. Without proper management and counseling, this can lead to higher levels of anxiety and a greater risk of depression leading to social, work-related, and personal problems.[130]

Discovering and developing other good qualities and things you have in your life will help you move your mind from the lost hair, and rediscover the inner strength that is not affected by hair loss.

The loss of your hair will awaken the truth of how temporary the things of this world are. You start to experience your own mortality. When I fully accepted my condition, I began to connect with the real me. I stopped relying on my outside appearance to prove who I really am. I now know I am okay with or without hair.

Both cold and hot seasons are quite challenging for people with hair loss, and one just needs to be aware of this and take the necessary care.

Finally, if you are starting to lose or have lost hair, begin to check for the underlying causes and if possible deal with them, to avoid other illnesses setting in at a late stage.

Thyroid Disease

Thyroid diseases or disorders are conditions that affect the thyroid gland, a butterfly-shaped gland in the front of the neck. The thyroid helps regulate numerous metabolic processes throughout the body. The thyroid gland uses iodine to produce important hormones in the body. Thyroid disease is a common problem that can cause symptoms because of over- or under-function of the thyroid gland. The thyroid gland is an essential organ for producing thyroid hormones, which maintain our body metabolism.

There are specific kinds of thyroid disorders that include:

- Hypothyroidism.
- Hyperthyroidism.
- Goiter.
- Thyroid nodules.
- Thyroid cancer.

Causes

According to the British Thyroid Foundation, the following are some of the causes:

- The primary cause of thyroid nodules and enlargement is unknown, but are more common in women than men.
- Women often develop thyroid enlargement during pregnancy and the menopause.
- Diffuse enlargement is often caused by autoimmune thyroid conditions such as Hashimoto's thyroiditis and Graves' disease and can be associated with a change in thyroid function.
- Iodine deficiency is the most common cause worldwide.

Types of thyroid nodules and swellings:

- Single thyroid nodule (solitary nodule).
- Multiple thyroid nodules (multinodular goiter)—sometimes caused by an over-active thyroid.
- Diffuse goiter—often found in Hashimoto's thyroiditis and Graves' disease (autoimmune thyroid disorders).
- Retrosternal goiter—the thyroid develops lower down behind the breastbone (often a multi-nodular goiter).

Complications associated with thyroid nodules include:

- **Problems swallowing or breathing.** Large nodules or a multinodular goiter—an enlargement of the thyroid gland containing several distinct nodules—can interfere with swallowing or breathing.
- **Hyperthyroidism.** Problems can occur when a nodule or goiter produces thyroid hormone, leading to hyperthyroidism. Hyperthyroidism can result in weight loss, muscle weakness, heat intolerance, and anxiousness or irritability, etc.

- **Problems associated with thyroid cancer.** If a thyroid nodule is cancerous, surgery is usually required. Generally, most or all of the thyroid gland is removed, after which you'll need to take thyroid hormone replacement therapy for the rest of your life.

Acid Reflux

Acid reflux or heartburn is a common condition that features a burning pain in the lower chest area and occurs when stomach acid flows back up into the food pipe. When this happens often (usually more than twice in a week), it is diagnosed as gastroesophageal reflux diseases which are due to lifestyle factors but sometimes due to some unpreventable factors.

Why One Needs to Treat and Control Acid Reflux or GERD

It is said that without treatment, GERD can lead to serious complications in the long term, including an increased risk of cancer as well as the following problems due to persistent exposure to stomach acid:

- **Esophagitis.** This is where the lining of the esophagus is inflamed, and can cause irritation, bleeding, and ulceration in some cases.
- **Strictures.** This is damage caused by stomach acid and can lead to scar development and difficulties swallowing, with food getting stuck as it travels down the esophagus.
- **Barrett's esophagus.** This is a severe complication where repeated exposure to stomach acid can cause changes in the cells and tissues lining the throat with the potential to develop into cancer cells.

Both esophagitis and Barrett's esophagus are associated with a higher risk of cancer.[131]

The following groups of foods and habits have been linked to acid reflux:

- Caffeine.
- Alcohol.
- A high intake of table salt.
- A diet low in dietary fiber.
- Eating large meals.
- Lying down within 2 to 3 hours of eating a meal.
- Consuming chocolate, carbonated drinks, and acidic juices.

A recent study (September 7, 2017) suggests that dietary choices may be as effective as using proton pump inhibitors (PPIs) in treating acid reflux.[132]

Acid reflux or GERD is a widespread problem with a number of people and going on my own experience, eliminating hurting food is very important even though one may be on medication. Personally, through the advice of a consultant, I was told it is a good idea to control the acid with proton pump inhibitors, and though I regularly take medication, I rely heavily on my dietary choices and lifestyle.

Drinking or sipping water often ensures any acid is washed away. I minimize acidic and spicy foods. Though fruits are great, there are some acidic fruits, such as oranges, clementines, tomatoes, etc. that I avoid in order to manage this problem. *Eating Right for Your Blood Type*[133] is a helpful book in trying to determine which foods can be hurting, and though the book doesn't help everyone, it was a good starting point for me. Fried foods and some oils can make the problem flare up. Different people react differently to different types of food, and hence you need to do your own checks to identify the foods that really hurt you. Once you have identified them, it is imperative to keep away from these foods.

The other useful information that really helped me is food combination. Vegetables seem to be a good combination with all food groups, while fruits are best eaten separately from other foods on an empty stomach and preferably a few minutes before meals.

Diabetes

Diabetes is a disease in which the body's ability to produce or respond to the hormone insulin is impaired, resulting in abnormal metabolism of carbohydrates and elevated levels of glucose in the blood.

According to Diabetes UK, diabetes is a serious life-long health condition that occurs when the amount of glucose (sugar) in the blood is too high because the body can't use it properly. If left untreated, high blood glucose levels can cause serious health complications.

I have witnessed several people suffering from diabetes, mainly type 2, including my mother and other close relatives and friends. Unlike cardiovascular diseases, diabetes may show some pre-symptoms and can be easily managed with diet as well as with medication. Due to lack of knowledge of the early symptoms, some people do not seek medical attention early enough, and hence it is discovered quite late when a lot of damage has already taken place in the body.

There is no definite way to know if you have diabetes without undergoing blood tests to determine your blood glucose levels. Diabetes is a risk factor for heart and kidney diseases and needs to be kept under control to avoid other organs being affected.

Glucose

Glucose is a simple sugar found in food and is an essential nutrient that provides energy for the proper functioning of the body cells. Carbohydrates are broken down in the small intestine, and the glucose in digested food is then absorbed by the intestinal cells into the bloodstream and is carried by the blood to all the cells in the body where it is utilized. For glucose to enter the cells, it will need insulin to help transport it into cells. Sometimes the cells develop insulin resistance and are unable to utilize the glucose, resulting in an increase of sugar in the bloodstream. The abundant, unutilized glucose is excreted in the urine.

Insulin

Insulin is a hormone that is produced by specialized cells of the pancreas. It helps glucose enter the cells and regulates the level of glucose in the body. For people with diabetes, the insulin is either absent, or relatively insufficient for the body's needs, or the body is unable to use it properly, and all these cause an increase of glucose in the blood, a condition known as hyperglycemia.

The Relationship Between Glucose and Insulin

The amount of glucose in the blood is controlled by the insulin hormone that is produced in the pancreas. The insulin transports glucose out of the blood and into cells where it is broken down to give energy. However, when one has diabetes, this process is hindered either because the insulin is not being produced, is not enough or does not work correctly.

There are Two Main Types of Diabetes: Type 1 and Type 2

Type 1 diabetes is an autoimmune condition where the immune system attacks and destroys insulin-producing cells in the pancreas, meaning no insulin is produced. This causes glucose to quickly rise in the blood. This causes diabetes by leaving the body without enough insulin to function normally.

In type 2 diabetes, the body doesn't make enough insulin, or the insulin it produces doesn't work properly, meaning glucose builds up in the blood. Experts say it is caused by a complex interplay of genetic and environmental factors.

Risk factors for type 2 diabetes and prediabetes are many. Often, the most overwhelming factor is a family history of type 2 diabetes. The following can raise risks of developing type 2 diabetes:

- Being obese or overweight.
- Living a sedentary lifestyle.
- Increasing age.
- Bad diet.
- High blood pressure.
- Elevated levels of triglycerides and low levels of "good" cholesterol (HDL).
- Polycystic ovary syndrome.
- Impaired glucose tolerance.
- Insulin resistance.
- Gestational diabetes during a pregnancy.
- Ethnic background. Some ethnic backgrounds are at a higher risk than others. Probably because of the diet and lifestyle choices of such groups of people.

There are no specific diabetes causes, but according to Diabetes UK the following triggers may be involved:

- Viral or bacterial infection.
- Chemical toxins within food.
- Unidentified component causing an autoimmune reaction.

Symptoms of Diabetes

According to most studies and NHS, some people with type 2 diabetes may not be aware or suspect that they have a serious condition because the symptoms do not initially make you feel unwell.

Symptoms of type 1 and type 2 diabetes include:

- Increased urine output especially at night.
- Excessive thirst.
- Unexplained weight loss.
- Hunger.
- Tiredness.
- Skin problems.
- Slow healing wounds.
- Yeast infections.
- Tingling or numbness in the feet or toes.

Other symptoms manifest as the disease progresses with time such as the inability to see clearly.

In type 2 diabetes, there is also a steady decline of beta cells that adds to the process of elevating blood sugars. Essentially, if someone is resistant to insulin, the body can, to some degree, increase production of insulin and overcome the level of resistance. With insulin resistance, the pancreas produces more and more insulin until the pancreas can no longer produce enough insulin for the body's demands, and then blood sugar rises. If production decreases and insulin cannot be released as vigorously, hyperglycemia develops.

Fruit and Diabetes

We know that everyone needs to eat more fruit and vegetables to support their health. In fact, current advice is to have at least 5 servings a day of fruit and vegetables. Indeed, according to a recent study by Imperial College London, the more the better and they even recommend 10 servings a day.

This recommendation is equally important to people with diabetes. Most people worry about the sugar content in fruit. However, the sugar content in fruit is natural and it's not the sugar people are advised against if eaten in the right portions. What should be reduced is added sugars in drinks, chocolates, cakes, and biscuits as well as in fruit juices and honey.

A diet of fruits and vegetables should not be taken instead of medicine. However, this type of diet provides our body with nutrients which the body uses to support its immune system and other systems, thereby enabling it to heal itself, even when one is on medication. I believe changing to this kind of diet is a win-win situation.

> Some people think plant-based, whole foods diet is extreme. Half a million people a year will have their chests opened up and a vein taken from their leg and sewn onto their coronary artery. Some people would call that extreme. (Dr. Caldwell Esselstyn, *No More Heart Attacks*)[134]

Cancer

As per the dictionary, cancer is a disease caused by an uncontrolled division of abnormal cells in a part of the body or a malignant growth or tumor resulting from an uncontrolled division of cells.

Cancer is a disease that has affected people all over the world either directly or indirectly. Almost everyone knows somebody whose life has been claimed by this disease, be it a relative, a neighbor, a colleague or a friend. Since this is a potentially deadly disease, I would encourage readers to get medical advice from a doctor urgently if they think they are suffering from this problem.

Though some victims of cancer eventually lose the battle to the diseases we have survivors as well, I believe it is not very clear why this is the case.

As mentioned in chapter 2, the primary causes of many diseases are toxicity, nutrition deficiency, nutrition overload leading to obesity, sedentary lifestyle, acidity, stress, etc., and it has been suggested that cancer is no exception though the real cause is not fully known. There is not enough evidence to prove that diet and change of lifestyle can heal people who are suffering from cancer, but a healthy diet may support their healing even as they go through treatment.

Other Diseases

Dementia, arthritis, celiac diseases, Crohns, rheumatism, arthritis, and acid reflux are also among many illnesses that are affecting many people all over the world. The medical world is doing the best they can to help humanity reduce their suffering. Our part is to assist this process by taking care of our health individually as we improve on our diets and lifestyle and that is the purpose of this book.

Chapter 14: Weight loss and Management

Weight was one area I struggled with for many years and though I may not have fully reached my goal, I know I have seen a significant improvement since I started to change the way I do things.

If you follow the ideas and diet recommended in this book, it will eventually lead to weight loss. If this leads to a consistent lifestyle change, it will ultimately bring permanent benefits.

There are many ways of losing weight and managing it depending on the strategy one uses. We will lose weight if we burn more calories than we consume. However, there are many ways of achieving this. I will not discuss other methods but one which I applied and gave me success and also the one recommended in these books, derived from the suggestions in the *Essene Gospel of Peace Book 1.*

How to Lose Weight and Keep it Away

It is imperative to have some understanding as to why one has put on weight even before trying to lose it. Being overweight or obese is about imbalance. It's a lack of balance between what one is eating and what one is burning. If you eat more than you burn you gain weight. What is weight? When we say we want to lose weight what are we talking about? Put simply, when people want to lose weight, it's not muscles and bones that they want to lose, but fat. How does fat in our bodies come about? When we consume more calories than the body is using, the excess calories are eventually changed to fat. Other sources of body fat are oils, fats, butter, etc.

The only way to get that fat off is to eat less and exercise more.[135]

We know that in the majority of cases excess calorific food is the cause of being overweight. To reverse this excess, we must check our diets and see where we are going wrong. One major step is to reduce your calorie intake. Reducing portion sizes will support your journey to weight loss. However, this must be done wisely to ensure that the body is still getting the essential nutrients it needs for its normal bodily functions. Also, as we have discussed in this book, the type of food we eat can either support weight loss or gain. People are different, and people gain weight due to various reasons such as excess calories, and lack of exercise, etc. Therefore, before thinking about how to lose weight, we need to ask ourselves why we put on weight. Only then will we be able to make permanent changes, by tackling the root cause.

I found this quote by the Duke of Sussex in *The Telegraph* which I think we can apply to our challenges with weight:

> I have seen time and time again, through my work with young people from across the Commonwealth, that today's generation understands something very important: that to tackle a big issue, you need to focus on the root causes of the challenge, not its symptoms. [136]

Though the above was said in relation to other social problems, the same can be said regarding obesity.

Things to observe:

- The diet recommended is a plant-based diet which should be at least 60% raw, the use of processed foods and animal products such as meat is not recommended, but some people use raw milk and eggs, while most on the whole plant-based diet avoid all animal products.
- Planning ahead and being thoughtful about what you want to achieve.

One will never succeed in any project if there is no prior planning. To change one's diet and lifestyle, one has to plan ahead the food they will eat and the physical activities they will get involved with. Start with clearing your fridge and drawers of all the fatty, processed, and sugary foods. Then make a list of the things you need to buy that will support you on a weekly basis. Think about your lunches, breakfasts, dinners, and snacks, and have meal plans to help you in this process. Going by the recommendations in this book, your food choices will be around fruits (such as apples, pineapples, papaya, mangoes, bananas, grapes, nectarines, berries etc.), vegetables (such as cucumbers, courgettes, spinach, kale, lettuce, celery, avocados, tomatoes, parsnip, carrots, cabbage, green beans, peas etc.), carbohydrates and starches (such as brown rice, potatoes, corn, quinoa, wheat, buckwheat, sweet potatoes, and many more), and for protein foods you have a selection of seeds, such as sesame, sunflower, lentils, broccoli, beans, legumes, soya and soya products, nuts such as almonds, peanuts, walnuts, etc., plus raw milk for those who still take milk. Alternative plant-based milks include hazelnut, almond, soya, hemp coconut, etc. Plan your meals bearing in mind the calorific content of the food. Your meals should be based on fruits, vegetables, and carbohydrates with proteins and dairy in small portions. If you can remember the previous topics, then you will recall that starches are not fattening if eaten in the right amounts and without adding oil to them.

Understanding Food and How the Body Works

For the benefit of calorie restriction and weight management, the first meal should be around noon, allowing 16–18 hours between your last and first meal.

Eating the first meal around 12 noon is helpful because it will give the body a chance to make use of the excess glycogen and fats. Dr. Mark Mattson, chief of the Laboratory of Neuroscience at the National Institute of Aging, says it takes about 10–12 hours for the body to deplete the glycogen from the liver before it starts using the stored fat (or earlier if one is exercising). Hence if one desires to lose weight, intermittent fasting is a great tool. *"Eat only when the sun is highest in the heavens, and again when it is set" (Essene Gospel of Peace Book 1).*[137] I know that many people regard breakfast as all-important. However, the method being proposed by the writer is where breakfast is taken later in the day not early in the morning, one can call it breakfast or first meal. However, in between, one can have drinks, teas, or green juices with low calories to ensure that we are not hindering the use of stored glycogen.

Exercise or Physical Activity

For all which has life does move (*Essene Gospel of Peace Book 1*)

One will need at least a minimum of 30 minutes or more of exercise for 6 days. This can be achieved by walking, cycling or going to the gym or any other activity that you are able to follow for at least 30 minutes. The UK government recommends a minimum of 150 minutes per week.

To maintain a healthy weight and avoid becoming overweight, energy from food needs to balance with the amount of energy burnt by the body during exercise or daily work. However, if we continue to consume more calories than we burn we will gain weight and become obese.

Please refer to the section about exercise in this book. However, for this section, we need to remember that burning more than we are taking will ensure you are on the journey towards losing weight.

Regular and Occasional Fasting

As I said earlier, I recommend eating 6 days and fasting 1 day a week. As much as this is for spiritual reasons, it is also a useful tool in helping balance out any excess eating during the week. Currently, there is a popular eating plan 5:2 whereby one eats 5 days and fasts for 2 days by consuming about 500 calories for women and 600 calories for men. This is a comfortable way of fasting, but it has excellent results as reported by Dr. Michael Mosley.[138]

Consistency and Persistence

Perseverance and repetition will make one form a habit; one has to repeat over and over again the methods that are giving them success choosing a healthy diet becomes a habit.

Change Diet and Lifestyle

It is not wise to wake up and decide you want to change without first incorporating your mind into the programme. Make up your mind on what you want to achieve, where you are, and where you want to go. Plan the food you want to be eating after the plan, make sure the food is balanced and is based on fruits, vegetables, and carbohydrates PLUS protein and dairy in smaller amounts. Any promise of losing weight where there is no change in diet and lifestyle is misleading. The loss is temporary, and the weight will come back. The other myth that I had lived with for a long time is that starch makes you add weight. It does not when eaten without adding oil and in the right portions, and it makes the food enjoyable. One needs to just take the right amount of protein and not excess. I think the majority of people take more than their daily requirement, which the recommended amount in the UK is approximately 45 grams for women and 55 for men. Men and women in the UK eat about 45–55% more protein than they need each day, according to the National Diet and Nutrition Survey.[139]

Eating up to twice the current RNI for protein is generally thought to be safe, but nutritionist Dr. Helen Crawley says: "There is certainly no benefit to having very high protein intakes, and individuals who require high energy intakes for whatever reason should consider how to increase energy intake without increasing protein intakes excessively." There is contradictory research as to whether there is a health risk if one eats a high-protein diet. A study from the University of California suggests there is a link to certain diseases if one consumes more proteins while other research suggests that eating a protein-rich diet reduced the risk.[140]

Challenges

Since you can't live in isolation, the diets of the people around you will make your change difficult in the beginning. You may still need to prepare meals for others if you are a mum, wife, or chef, etc. and this may slow your intended change. Perseverance and talking to your family and friends may help you overcome these challenges. However, they can also oppose your new way of eating since they don't understand the reasons behind the change. Regardless of all these persevere and with time change will eventually come. Eating in social places can become challenging as well, but one can overcome this by carrying their own food. Some foods in the house may tempt you, and hence you need to learn how to deal with temptation or better still avoid the purchase of that particular food.

Making your lifestyle simple is key. Be concerned about the quality rather than quantity. Eat to live, and don't live to eat. Avoid eating out or takeaways whenever possible. It is fine to enjoy food when you are eating but eating to live a happy, healthy life is crucial for not just your health, but for the health of those around you. When one is sick, he doesn't only trouble himself but also his relatives and friends. Therefore, we all have a social responsibility to remind everyone around us of the need to live a healthy lifestyle.

I believe if you follow faithfully the above programme, you will experience a dramatic change in your life. It may take time before results begin to show, but they will eventually.

> Health is much more dependent on our habits and nutrition than on medicine.[141]

Chapter 15: Essene Diet in Brief

In summary, the diet recommended in the *Essene Gospel of Peace Book 1* which Rev. Abba Nazariah, DD, has called "The Jesus Diet," should ideally be:

- A raw plant-based diet or a raw food vegetarian diet, whereby the foods are consumed uncooked or slightly cooked so that the nutrients are not destroyed; in other words, "living foods." The food groups extensively mentioned include fruits, grains, seeds, and grasses of the field (all vegetables, plants good for eating, etc.).

- Animal milk is good; though bear in mind my discussion on pasteurized cow's milk, above.

- No meat should be consumed in the diet. Though unknown to many, Jesus stopped the killing of animals for sacrifice and flesh eating. Therefore, in this diet, eating of meat is not only considered unhealthy but wrong too.

- Less is better, and hence in this diet, people are advised to eat less frequently, and at most twice a day.

- The first meal of the day should be later from around 11am (as explained earlier in this book).

- Other recommendations include the use of water, slow eating, and proper chewing of food (to enable maximum absorption), and deep breathing while having meals.

- Jesus showed them how to cook bread in the sun without fire cooking, the famous 'Essene bread,' which involves first sprouting of wheat kennels, grinding it, preparing the wafers, and putting them in the sun for 'cooking.' This is only possible for people who live where the sun is always hot and hence people have come up with different ideas of how to cook the Essene bread. The idea behind is to avoid destruction of the nutrients with fire.

- Movement or physical exercise and regular fasting are also recommended in this diet.

- In this diet, I advise you feed the body for 6 days and take a break on the 7th day, a form intermittent fasting, where food should not be consumed and instead spend that time seeking the kingdom of God, this is definitely something we rarely do, but it appears it is good for our wellbeing.

Chapter 16: Change Can Happen to Anyone

Helpful Discourses by Luigi Cornaro, 1464—1566

Luigi Cornaro's story was one of the most fascinating I encountered in my journey towards health. It impacted my life significantly. Though he died many years ago, he wrote things down and so we can all benefit from his discourses.

When he was about 40 years old, Cornaro found himself exhausted and in poor health, a condition he attributed to a hedonistic lifestyle with excessive eating, drinking, and sexual licentiousness. At the advice of his doctors, he cured himself and having done that he continued to practice his new-found theory of self-control and moderation for the rest of his life. Without deviating from that path, he made up his mind to follow through.

He went on to live to the age of 102, according to some records, but not because he had good genes. In fact, he was sick and almost dying until a physician helped to recover his health. Luigi Cornaro's story is inspiring because though almost dying at 40 he went on to live for many years and not only living but also, he was strong and healthy and able to write till very late in life.

> This should be the desire for anyone longing to live for many years. And I further maintain that dying in the manner I expect is not really death but a passage of the soul from this earthly life to a celestial immortal, and infinitely perfect existence. Whence it is that I enjoy two lives and the thought of terminating this earthly life gives me no concern, for I know that I have a glorious and immortal life before me. I expect to pass away quietly and peacefully, and my present condition insures this to me, though I have attained this great age I am hearty and content, eating with good appetite and sleeping soundly. (*The Essene Science of Fasting*)[142]

As written by Antonio Maria Grazia, "He then disposed himself with dignity, and closing his eyes as if in slumber, gave a gentle sigh and expired."[143] It is recorded that this is precisely what happened; the soul just left the body while he was seated. This should be everyone's goal; however, it's not achieved without a total change of the way we do things, what, how and when to eat, and the status of our mind and emotions (feelings).

Whereas, I, in my old age, praise to the Almighty, am exempt from these torments; from the first, because I cannot fall sick, having removed all the cause of illness by my regularity and moderation; from the other, that of death, because from so many years' experience, I have learned to obey reason; whereas, I not only think it a great folly to fear that which cannot be avoided, but likewise firmly expect some consolation from the grace of Jesus Christ, when I arrive at that period. (Luigi Cornaro, *How to Live 100 Years*)[144]

Cornaro maintained that longevity was desirable and "God wills it." He rejected ascetics who believed man must suffer in this life to attain salvation in the next, arguing that there was no reason he could not enjoy both an earthly existence and his heavenly one. In addition, he rejected the conventional wisdom that old age was a period of misery and decay. He wrote:

Some sensual unthinking persons affirm that a long life is no great blessing and that the state of a man, who has passed his seventy-fifth year, cannot really be called life; but this is wrong, as I shall fully prove; and it is my sincere wish, that all men would endeavor to attain my age, that they might enjoy that period of life, which of all others is most desirable. (Luigi Cornaro, *The Art of Living Long*)[145]

He also commented that, at the age of 83, his health was good, he could perform most functions unassisted, and he had a wide circle of younger friends and correspondents. Cornaro also firmly condemned those with a live-fast-and-die-young mentality, stating that, "They don't stop and consider the virtue of ten more years of active life, at a point where we've reached a high point of experience and wisdom, two things that can only be honed with time." (*Discourse of Sober Life*)[146]

My Lord, to begin, I must tell you, that being now at the age of ninety-one, I am sounder and heartier than ever, much to the amazement of those who know me. I, who can account for it, am bound to show that a man can enjoy a terrestrial paradise after eighty; but it is not to be obtained, except by strict temperance in food and drink, virtues acceptable to God and friends to reason. (*Third Discourse*)[147]

It follows, therefore, that it is impossible to be a perfect physician to another. A man cannot have a better guide than himself, nor any physic better than a regular life. I do not, however, mean that for the knowledge and cure of such disorders as befall those who live an irregular life there is no occasion for a physician and that his assistance ought to be slighted; such persons should at once call in medical aid, in case of sickness.

But, for the bare purpose of keeping ourselves in good health, I am of the opinion that we should consider this regular life as our physician, since it preserves men, even those of a weak constitution, in health; makes them live sound and hearty, to the age of one hundred and upward, and prevents their dying of sickness, or through the corruption of their humors, but merely by the natural decay, which at the last must come to all. These things, however, are discovered but by a FEW, for men, for the most part, are sensual and intemperate, and love to satisfy their appetites, and to commit every excess; and, by way of apology, say that they prefer a short and self-indulgent life, to a long and self-denying one, not knowing that those men are most truly happy who keep their appetites in subjection. (Luigi Cornaro, *How to Live 100 Years*).[148]

What I learned from Luigi Cornaro, is that if we start to assist our bodies to heal, they eventually will. He believed that the body could cure itself if an individual corrected his daily habits of eating and living. One of the methods he used is what we today call calorie control—but to him, it was living a sober life, or sobriety, where his food and drink intake was restricted.

This sobriety, or self-control/self-restraint, is reduced to two things, quality and quantity. The first consists in avoiding food or drinks which are found to disagree with the stomach. The second, to avoid taking more than the stomach can easily digest.

He fasted often or practiced what we now call intermittent fasting because he ate little and at set times. He learned to respect his body and decided to help other human beings that would come after him by penning his journals. He prayed and hoped for eternal life and understood the essence of the soul and its final journal to eternity. He stopped worrying about death and endeavored to live his life the best way he could. Though Cornaro started his health journey when he was younger than me, I was fascinated by his life, and I thought maybe even for me, I can at least try reducing some of the damage that I have already done to my body. He also made me see the importance of writing; you help other people apart from yourself. Many people may not have the desire or inspiration to look for information, but when you write it down for them, you may save their lives, and this fulfills a great part of our responsibility to help our fellow human beings.[149]

Chapter 17: Conclusions

Good health is everyone's dream, and no one plans to be sick. However, as time passes by, we all get some health issues here and there, some mild and others serious. The underlying causes of diseases are various, and while sometimes we put emphasis on the symptoms, it is vital to go deeper and check for the hidden causes of disease. Diseases do not just appear, but little by little, the wrongs we do to our bodies eventually become major diseases.

The purpose of a raw plant-based diet is to help us feed our bodies with living food that is not damaged, denatured or deprived of nutrients. The consequences of feeding our bodies with food that is not constitutionally right and is devoid of nutrients eventually show up, and we get sick. The question is whether it is possible to go back to the original diet that God intended for humanity? I hope by reading this book, you will start to ask yourself some hard questions. The information in the *Essene Gospel of Peace* (mainly Book 1) enabled me to get some answers to some of the questions which were resonating in my mind relating to food. The Essenes were a unique group of people that appeared to have been a more spiritual sect than any other group during the time of Jesus. The diet they finally decided to follow, which can be called *The Essene Diet*, was initially taught to them by Jesus and they were dumbfounded when they heard of it for the first time.

Fasting is a widely used method all over the world, and it can help us recover our health. Jesus said, "When you fast," which shows he expected His disciples to fast regularly, this is beneficial both spiritually and physically. Health involves our mind, body, and spirit, the trinity of health; our whole being must be involved to give us complete health.

In many parts of the world, people struggle to keep their weight down, and though sometimes genetics can be blamed, it is true that the right diet, the correct amount of food together with physical exercise, can help one achieve or significantly improve on their weight goals.

In the *Gospel of Thomas*, Jesus is reported to have said, "If the flesh came into being because of the spirit, it is amazing, but if the spirit came into being because of the body, it's even more amazing. I am amazed, though at how such great wealth has settled into such poverty."[150]

The physical body we see is temporary and will one day pass away. However, we all have a responsibility to take care of it so that it does not impede or stop us from achieving our purposes on Earth because of the diseases and issues it has to deal with.

I believe that some of the conditions I have mentioned, such as cardiovascular diseases, autoimmune diseases, Alopecia Universalis, acid reflux, thyroid, diabetes, cancer, dementia, etc. can be avoided, or controlled if one would drastically change their diet and lifestyle early enough when the body is still strong. Nevertheless, regardless of where one is in life, one can still make changes, it is never too late to try. The body will start to rebuild itself, and somehow it knows what to do if you give it the material it needs.

> I continue to be amazed by our bodies' ability for self-repair.... Our bodies want to be healthy if we would just let them. That's what these new research articles are showing: Even after years of beating yourself up with a horrible diet, your body can reverse the damage, open back up the arteries-even reverse the progression of some cancers. Amazing! So, it's never too late to start exercising, never too late to stop smoking and never too late to start eating healthier. (*Michael Greger MD*)[151]

Currently, the Western diet has been blamed for many health problems However it is everyone's responsibility to change their diet and lifestyle to be able to escape or reduce some of the onslaughts of disease made worse by the modern diet.

> No one escapes in the end. Eventually, the traditional Western diet guarantees some form of disease in all of the people. While it may not be heart disease now, eventually it will be a form of illness or hypertension, diabetes, stroke, obesity, gall stones, diverticulitis, rheumatoid arthritis, lupus, multiple sclerosis, or a greater likelihood of breast, prostate, colon, ovarian, and uterine cancers. Even erectile dysfunction and dementia. BUT there is something that you can do now to stop the cascading events that occur in the body and lead to disease and conditions as mentioned above. You can change your diet and begin safeguarding your health for the future. (*Dr. Esselstyn*)[152]

The poem I wrote for my mother (see the next section) reminded me of the many things that mother nature gives to us freely, which we take for granted.

Poem to My Mother

Wish

If only my mother knew that health was her greatest wealth, and it was determined largely by her own action, probably she would have faced life differently.

If only my mother knew that giving me that apple, plum or berry, was good enough food, she would not have felt the need to go seeking the butcher's provision to give her children the delicacies she thought would do us good.

If only my mother knew how blessed she was to be able to grow all those organic vegetables with little effort. The soil so rich and loamy with organic manure from the many animals she kept.

If only my mother knew that the food she grew had already been pre-cooked by the sun and needed not much cooking if any at all. She would have enjoyed life without struggles of so many hours of smoke trying to put food on the table.

If only my mother knew the corn and the potatoes she grew were good food for her children, all she needed to do was to add fruit and vegetables, what a life she would have led.

If only my mother knew how blessed she was to be able to grow those garden peas, runner beans, cabbages, kales, pumpkins, spring onions, potatoes, sweet potatoes, arrow roots, carrot, passion fruits, and many more, without watering or pesticides. She would have just spent more time praising her Heavenly Father for His great provision.

If only my mother knew how much mother nature had favored her with all she needed to feed her children, she would have considered herself a blessed woman, in spite of being short of money.

If only my mother knew the organic raw milk she got from her animals was a complete food in its natural form, she would have not spent hours destroying, denaturing or reducing its nutrients through boiling.

If only my mother knew how blessed she was to have a spring on her farm and to be able to get fresh water from the springs. If only she could have opened her eyes to see the millions in the vicinity without water, then she would have considered herself lucky.

If only my mother knew that we had enough good food. She would not have gone to the shops to bring meat, and other processed foods that she thought were better for us.

If only my mother knew she would have been more confident in using what was available to her, she would have treasured it as gold; she would have educated me and her other children, and given us more knowledge to use.

History

Yes, we didn't have much money, but we had enough food to eat and to give away. We never slept hungry not even one day. One may ask why we didn't turn our produce to money, but with no transport and miles of walking, you could not easily transport your produce to the market.

I still remember how colorful our Christmas was, the sun was bright, new clothes, and ripe plums all over the place. Those plums trees of many different varieties made Christmas so beautiful. And those fruit trees with branches hanging with abundant fruits, ah, me and my sister could just sit underneath their shade and eat until we couldn't eat anymore. It's funny how we never got fed up with those fruits.

If only I could stand there and watch as my grandfather harvested raw honey from our beehive. Oh, how we enjoyed the honey in its honeycomb. I did not know how privileged we were to experience that. We would not have moved to the city with the idea that our food was inferior; we would not have gone to embrace foreign foods while abandoning ours. We exchanged our natural food for fried rice, pilau, chapati made with white flour, cornmeal from refined maize flour.

We started frying almost everything. Our specials were chips, sausages, hot dogs, burgers, sausage rolls, spring chicken, and meat on a daily basis. Now our milk was no longer direct from the animals; it was now in special bottles and packets from the supermarket. Oh, how advanced we had become!

City life was far better than the farm life; everything was readily available, and we never needed to farm to get food if we had money to buy what we needed. All this was because of our lack of knowledge. Mother, you never spoke or knew how superior your food was; you got carried away. You were glad to come to the city and eat of our delicacies.

We were blessed to be able to live on a farm with so many trees producing fresh oxygen for us, the sun rose us early in the morning, and the sunsets were a wonder to see. At night we would enjoy the sight of the beautiful stars in the sky with no worries in the world except one.

We thought ours was not good enough; we felt God was unfair to us, and we looked forward to a life in the city. With not enough money or nice housing, we ate the village food, but all the while wanting the city life, the housing, the electricity, and running water. We thought life had denied us good things and so we went looking for them. Yes, we got some of those things we desired, but we also left behind some of mother nature's gifts. We exchanged her food for that which is no food, and today we regret our actions.

If only I could rewind time and get to live with Mum on our old farm again, endowed with my current knowledge. I would access that pure organic milk that we used to get from grass-fed animals that were happy to graze walking up and down the hills, drinking clean water directly from the spring and from the Irate river next to the Aberdare's forests where I would swim and immerse myself countless times again.

Oh, if only my mother knew how blessed she was! If only she taught me, probably I would have listened, and perhaps this book would be talking about something else.

Since my mum left, I have struggled with some health issues, and now I know a good diet, especially the one we had when growing up, would have kept my body in a better condition.

If only we stayed on our vegetables, fruit, corn, peas, beans, kale, potatoes, and sweet potatoes; if we just used raw milk like that which we produced. If just we maintained those long-distance walks like we used to; then the troubles of health would not have been my portion.

If only meat remained scarce like when we were growing up; in fact, if only no animal was killed for meat. I know we rarely killed our own animals, nevertheless we occasionally visited the butcher.

If only mum had stopped using animal fat for frying food because it was and is deadly as I know it today. If only she knew more about nutrition, she would not have gotten diabetes because she had done so well in other areas.

If only my grandmother taught her—if only she knew and taught me to teach my children. A ripple effect would have been created, and probably we would have been some of the healthiest people in the world. Perhaps some of her adorable children would not have departed from this life prematurely. I know they never grew on the farm, but still, she would have mentioned to them early enough about her superior foods whenever she had the opportunity to.

I still remember her pain when her beloved son was no more and then as if that was not enough, she experienced again the departure of her daughter, who was like her "mother" and anchor. They both meant the world to her. It was scary to all of us, we felt left alone, but God's grace was enough for us, and He enabled us to cope even we were faced with another similar loss later.

If only my mother knew, probably she would have been around to see my children grow and those of her other children. They did not enjoy her love, smile, and laughter. Oh, how I wish the clocks could rewind, and I start all over again.

Present

I'm trying to learn a bit of nutrition now, with a change in diet and lifestyle, a bit late but better late than never.

I'm trying to incorporate some of my childhood foods and ways of living. Though I cannot get everything as pure as it was then, I'm trying.

I now live in a city where one can get anything if they can afford it. When my children were babies, I did not have any really good information on food and the way it should be eaten.

Now they are big, and I hope I will be able to tell them about the goodness that we consumed, the spring water we drank, the organic milk, fruit trees, the wild berries, and all manner of herbs. Green leafy vegetables grew without much effort. The beautiful sunshine that was never deadly hot for us. The walking that kept us healthy, yet we did not know how amazing that was for our body; it also gave us the stamina to work long hours.

Mother nature knew what we needed and gave us exactly that. But due to lack of knowledge, we thought she gave us inferior foods, and we desired the food made by man and despised her food, we developed new taste buds.

Now, wherever we find ourselves, we need to open our eyes and see what mother nature has for us there. It's probably enough and we need not panic seeking alternatives. We can use what the land produces, and we will be amazed by how enough it is.

Oh, my tears roll down for all the years I have lived in ignorance. Oh, how blind I have been, oh, how blind! My eyes are starting to see better, but my will to do the right thing is still weak, I have been prodigal for too long, but I'm getting there.

They say it's better late than never and probably I'm blessed to know some of these things when I have breath with me. Perhaps somebody will learn from me and pass it on to somebody else. Hopefully, my children will not repeat this poem.

It's not all lost; my mother introduced me to her Saviour, my Saviour Jesus Christ. There is no greater legacy than that. My mother read Bible stories to my sister and me every night. She taught us a lot that pertains to life; her voice is a constant in my life. I still remember her nightly prayers and the faith she introduced us to keep us going strong.

May my Mum rest in eternal peace

About the Author

Florence W. Mabwa works at Phoenix Mortgages & Financial Services as a Financial Consultant (Mortgages & Protection). In addition to her other training, she has also trained in the following courses which give her a deeper understanding in the areas of diet and nutrition: Diet Specialist course (Accredited by Association for Nutrition, AFN), Nutrition & Health Eating, Nutrition for Weight Loss by High-Speed Training. Florence, on a voluntary basis, facilitates events that talks about diet and healthy lifestyle.

Her goal is to enlighten others in matters relating to their diet and lifestyle choice, that includes whole plant-based nutrition together with an active lifestyle as inspired by the *Essene Gospel of Peace Book 1*

Bibliography

Adamo, Dr. P. J. D., *Eat Right for your Type.*

Allen, James, *As a Man Thinketh.*

Barber, G and F. Borrelli, *The Insync Diet.*

Bowles, Jeff T., *The Miraculous Results of Vitamin D3*, 2010.

Bragg, Paul C & Patricia, *The Miracle of Fasting.*

Bragg, Paul C, *Build Powerful Nerve Force.*

Campbell, T. C., *Folks & Knives.*

Cornaro, Luigi, *How to Live to 100 Years.*

Cornaro, Luigi, *The Art of Living Long*, 1903.

Cornaro, Luigi, *Discourses on Sober Life.*

Carper, J., *Food Your Miracle Medicine,* 1993.

Ehret, Prof. Arnold, *Physical Fitness Thru a Superior Diet, Fasting and Dietetics.*

Ehret, Prof. Arnold, *The Mucusless Diet Healing System*, 2013.

Howel, Dr. Edward, *Enzyme Nutrition, The Food Enzyme.*

Ignarro, Dr. J. Louis, *No More Heart Diseases*, 2008.

Mcdoughal J. A. and Mary Mcdoughal, *The Starch Solution*, 2012.

Meyer, M. W., *The Nag Hammadi Scriptures*, International Edition 2009.

Pessin, Donna, *Unique Healing*, 2011.

Porter, C. S., *Milk Diet as a Remedy for Chronic Diseases*, 2011.

Sinclair, Upton, *The Fasting Cure,* original edition 1911 re-printed.

Szekely, E. D, *The Essene Gospel of Peace 1*, London 1937.

Szekely, E. D, *The Gospel of Essenes Book 2 and 3,* 1986.

Wheater, Caroline, *Juicing for Health.*

Vazquez, M., *Alopecia & Wellness.*

Yakos, Marvin, *Prevent Life Decay*, 2003.

Endnotes

[1] Dr. Edward Howel, *Enzyme Nutrition*. Avery Publishing 1985.

[2] See *Essene Gospel of Peace*, Complete 4 books in one volume, 145–149.

[3] Lars Muhlmessiah, *The Law of Light*. Watkins Publishing, 2014.

[4] The *Essene Gospel Of Peace Book 1*, 7.

[5] Luigi Cornaro, *The Art of Living Long*. Kessinger Publishing, 2010.

[6] Arnold Ehret, *The Mucusless Diet Healing System*. Ehret Literature Publishing, 1994.

[7] Luigi Cornaro, *The Art of Living Long*. Kessinger Publishing, 2010.

[8] Arnold Ehret, *The Mucusless Diet Healing System*. Ehret Literature Publishing, 1994.

[9] According to Dr Ben Kim DC (http:// drbenkim.com/full-body-cleanse.htm), also author of *7 Keys to Overcoming Autoimmune Illness*, we have in other words two types of toxins, metabolic OR endogenous toxins and environmental OR exogenous toxins.

[10] http://drbenkim.com/

[11] Source Acidosis and Alkalosis (5 March 2014). labtestsonline.org/understanding/conditions/acidosis

[12] https://healthprep.com/conditions/5-common-symptoms-of-inflammatory-disease

[13] https://www.cancerresearchuk.org

[14] https://www.livescience.com

[15] (http://www.cancer.gov/cancertopics/wyntk/non-hodgkin-lymphoma

[16] https://www.livescience.com/26983-lymphatic-system.html, February 20, 2018

[17] According to the National Lymphadema Network.

[18] azquotes.com

[19] Luigi Cornaro, *The Art of Living Long*. Kessinger Publishing, 2010.

[20] azquotes.com

[21] *Essene Gospel of Peace Book 1*, 14.

[22] Luigi Cornaro, *The Art of Living Long*. Kessinger Publishing, 2010.

[23] Luigi Cornaro. *How to Live 100 Years*. Kessinger Publishing, 2010.

[24] R. Berger. Agnes Karll Schwest Krankenpfleger. 1968 Jul 22(7):315.

[25] drbenkim.com.

[26] https://thefastdiet.co.uk/

[27] E. B. Szekely, *The Essene Science of Fasting and the Art of Sobriety*. IBS, 1981.

[28] E. B. Szekely, *The Essene Science of Fasting and the Art of Sobriety*. IBS, 1981.

[29] *Essene Gospel of Peace Book 1*, 28.

[30] *Essene Gospel of Peace Book 1*, 32.

[31] E. B. Szekely, *The Essene Science of Fasting and the Art of Sobriety*. IBS, 1981.

[32] Paul and Patricia Bragg, *The Miracle of Fasting*. Health Science, 2015.

[33] https://www.buchinger.de/en/buchinger-therapeutic-fasting/the-original-method/

[34] https://www.bbc.co.uk/news/health-44005092

[35] https://www.drberg.com/blog/autophagy-and-intermittent-fasting

[36] *Essene Gospel of Peace Book 1*, 15.

[37] https://gerson.org/gerpress/the-gerson-therapy/

[38] *Essene Gospel of Peace Book 1*, 37.

[39] *Essene Gospel of Peace Book 1*, 41.

[40] draxe.com

[41] See for example https://www.nutristrategy.com

[42] https://www.ars.usda.gov/plains-area/gfnd/gfhnrc/docs/news-2013/dark-green-leafy-vegetables/

[43] http://www.hollandandbarrett.com/the-health-hub/go-green-boost-wellbeing/

[44] http://www.chm.bris.ac.uk/motm/chlorophyll/chlorophyll_h.htm by Paul May, University of Bristol. See also https://www.webmd.com/vitamins/ai/ingredientmono-712/chlorophyll

[45] "http://www.chm.bris.ac.uk/motm/chlorophyll/chlorophyll_h.htm"

[46] *Essene Gospel of Peace Book 1*, 43.

[47] https://www.fda.gov/food/resourcesforyou/consumers/ucm079516.htm

[48] https://thetruthaboutcancer.com/pasteurized-milk/

[49] https://www.theguardian.com, Tue 30 May 2017

[50] dr.axe.com.

[51] https://articles.mercola.com/sites/articles/archive/2018/10/16/why-is-raw-milk-illegal.aspx

[52] http://en.go-to-japan.jp/daisenguide

[53] *Essene Gospel of Peace Book 1*, 39.

[54] *Essene Gospel of Peace Book 1*, 36–37.

[55] Lars Muhlmessiah, *The Law of Light*. Watkins Publishing, 2014, 16.

[56] Gideon Jasper Richard Ouseley, *Gospel of the Holy Twelve*, 63.

[57] *Essene Gospel of Peace Book 1*, 42.

[58] Arnold Ehret, *The Mucusless Diet Healing System*. Ehret Literature Publishing, 1994.

[59] https://www.annualreviews.org/doi/10.1146/annurev-nutr-071816-064634 See also https://www.ncbi.nlm.nih.gov/pubmed/26135345

[60] https://nutritionstudies.org/author/mklaper/

[61] https://www.bbcgoodfood.com

[62] *Essene Gospel of Peace Book 1*, 42.

[63] These days, the year-round availability of everything from Peruvian asparagus to Dutch tomatoes is pretty much ubiquitous in UK supermarkets. www.the guardian.com of 12/08/2014.

[64] Paul and Patricia Bragg, *The Miracle of Fasting*. Health Science, 2015.

[65] *Essene Gospel of Peace Book 1*, 42.

[66] http://proverbicals.com

[67] Benjamin Franklin. *Rules of Health*.

[68] *Essene Gospel of Peace Book 1*, 45.

[69] *Essene Gospel of Peace Book 1*, 46.

[70] https://www.azquotes.com

[71] http://www.azquotes.com/quote/684366

[72] https://www.azquotes.com

[73] http://www.cooperinstitute.org

[74] http://www.cooperinstitute.org

[75] https://www.medicalnewstoday.com/articles/321846.php

[76] Notable-quotes.com

[77] *Essene Gospel of Peace Book 1*, 11.

[78] *Essene Gospel of Peace Book 1*, 28.

[79] Penn State researcher Barbara Rolls, PhD, author of *The Volumetrics Weight Control Plan*.

[80] https://www.webmd.com/diet/features/6-reasons-to-drink-water#1

[81] Harvard Health Publishing 13th April 2018.

[82] https://www.consciouslifestylemag.co

[83] http://ucsdnews.ucsd.edu/newsrel/health/08-07VitaminDKE-.asp

[84] https://www.medicaldaily.com/sun-exposure-vitamin-d-and-other-health-benefits-sunlight-246487.

[85] nhs.co.uk

[86] http://www.ncbi.nlm.nih.gov/pmc/articles/PMC2077351/

[87] http://medical-dictionary.thefreedictionary.com/nitric+oxide

[88] http://www.thelancet.com/aboutus

[89] In a study reported by Marianne Berwick, an epidemiology professor at the University of New Mexico, in the February 2005 *Journal of the National Cancer Institute.*

[90] https://www.bbcgoodfood.com/howto/guide/what-plant-based-diet

[91] https://www.bda.uk.com

[92] https://rawfoodlife.com/starting-raw-food/

[93] https://www.theguardian.com

[94] Jeff Novick, MS, RDN

[95] Arnold Ehret, *The Mucusless Diet Healing System.* Ehret Literature Publishing, 1994.

[96] https://www.healthyeating.org

[97] More on his work can be found on his website www. drmcdoughall.com

[98] Arnold Ehret, *The Mucusless Diet Healing System.* Ehret Literature Publishing, 1994, 57, 83.

[99] Paul Bragg, *Miracle of Fasting.*

[100] Wellness Bound Magazine, April 2004.

[101] To quicken in other words, refresh, revive, revitalize, activate or resuscitate etc.

[102] By Annette Larkins, a 75 years old lady.

[103] Essene Gospel of Peace Book 1, 40.

[104] Enzyme Nutrition, The Food Enzyme Concept by Dr Howard Howell.

[105] Dr Edward Howell, Enzyme Nutrition.

[106] Enzyme Nutrition by Dr Edward Howard.

[107] *Essene Gospel of Peace Book 1*, page 43.

[108] See studies by Dr Esselstyn, *No More Heart Attack*, and also www.forksoverknives.com

[109] http://www.msdmanuals.com

[110] Source: Wikipedia

[111] https://en.wikipedia.org/wiki/Genetic_disorders

[112] https://www.bhf.org.uk/heart-health/risk-factors

[113] https://www.onegreenplanet.org/news/watch-70-year-old-raw-vegan-looks-decades-younger

[114] Dr. Caldwell Esselstyn Jr as quoted on the documentary "Forks Over Knives."

[115] Michael Greger and Gene Stone, *How Not to Die.* Pan, 2017.

[116] https://www.telegraph.co.uk/foodanddrink/11552726/The-truth-about-sugar-in-fruit

[117] https://www.telegraph.co.uk/foodanddrink/11552726/The-truth-about-sugar-in-fruit-how-much-you-should-really-eat.htm

[118] More on his work can be found on https://nutritionstudies.org/about/dr-t-colin-campbell/

[119] http://www.dresselstyn.com/site/why-does-the-diet-eliminate-oil-entirely

[120] Dr Esselstyn, author of *No More Heart Attacks* also can be found in the above link.

[121] And also more on his website https://www.drmcdougall.com/

[122] https://en.wikipedia.org/wiki/Nitric_oxide#cite_note-pmid1361684-7

[123] https://www.ncbi.nlm.nih.gov/pubmed/15309199

[124] https://www.ncbi.nlm.nih.gov/pubmed/22240497

[125] https://www.diabetes.co.uk/autoimmune-diseases.htm

[126] http://www.healthywomen.org

[127] Dr.axe.com

[128] https://www.nhs.uk/conditions/leaky-gut-syndrome/

[129] https://rarediseases.info.nih.gov/diseases/614/alopecia-universalis

[130] /www.nhs.uk/hairloss

[131] https://www.medicalnewstoday.com/articles/146619.php

[132] https://jamanetwork.com/journals/jamaotolaryngology/article-abstract/2652893

[133] Dr Peter J. D. Adamo, *Eat Right For Your Type*. Penguin, 2003.

[134] Dr. Caldwell Esselstyn Jr quoted on the documentary "Forks Over Knives."

[135] Jack Lalanne quote, successstory.com

[136] 24/06/2018 by Telegraph.co.uk

[137] *Essene Gospel of Peace Book 1*, 42.

[138] https://www.sbs.com.au/food/article/2016/09/20/easy-health-hack-late-breakfast-michael-mosleys-secret-weapon.

[139] https://www.bbc.com/food/diets/should_you_worry_about_how_much_protein_you_eat

[140] http://www.bbc.co.uk/guides/z8899j6.

[141] John Lubback, www.statusmind.com

[142] E. B. Szekely, *The Essene Science of Fasting and the Art of Sobriety*. IBS, 1981.

[143] Luigi Cornaro, *The Art of Living Long*. Kessinger Publishing, 2010.

[144] Luigi Cornaro, *How to Live 100 Years*. Kessinger Publishing, 2010.

[145] Luigi Cornaro, *The Art of Living Long*. Kessinger Publishing, 2010.

[146] Luigi Cornaro, *Discourse of Sober Life*. Forgotten Books, 2018.

[147] Luigi Cornaro, *Discourse of Sober Life*. Forgotten Books, 2018.

[148] Luigi Cornaro, *How to Live 100 Years*. Kessinger Publishing, 2010.

[149] The above can be read in many of his discourses and in the book *How to Live Over 100 Years* by Luigi Cornaro.

[150] Gospel of Thomas in *The Secrets Teachings of Jesus Christ*, edited by Marvin Meyer. Random House, 1988. Pages 38–39.

[151] https://www.richroll.com

[152] http://www.DrEsselstyn.com